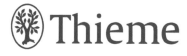

Fitness for the Pelvic Floor

Second Edition

Beate Carrière, PT, CIFK, CAPP
Private Practice
Lübeck, Germany

Dawn-Marie Ickes, PT, MPT, PhD, PMA-CPT
Associate Professor
Wellness Programming Coordinator
Mount Saint Mary's University
Los Angeles, CA, USA;
Director, MSMU Pilates Pro Bono Clinic
Los Angeles, CA, USA;
Private Practice, Evolve Integrative Wellness
Orange County, CA, USA

110 images

Thieme
Stuttgart • New York • Delhi • Rio de Janeiro

Library of Congress Cataloging-in-Publication Data is available with the publisher

Illustrator: Martin Hoffmann, Neu-Ulm, Germany

1st English edition, 2001
1st German edition, 2006
1st Korean edition, 2016

© 2024. Thieme. All rights reserved.

Georg Thieme Verlag KG
Rüdigerstrasse 14, 70469 Stuttgart, Germany
+49 [0]711 8931 421, customerservice@thieme.de

Cover design: © Thieme
Cover image source: © Thieme
Typesetting by Thomson Digital, India

Printed in Germany by Beltz Grafische Betriebe GmbH   5 4 3 2 1

DOI: 10.1055/b000000228

ISBN 978-3-13-242398-5

Also available as an e-book:
eISBN(PDF): 978-3-13-242400-5
eISBN(epub): 978-3-13-258112-8

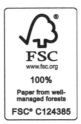

FSC
www.fsc.org
100%
Paper from well-managed forests
FSC® C124385

Contents

Videos

Foreword

As a physician involved in the evaluation and treatment of pelvic floor disorders, I am very impressed with the second edition of *Fitness for the Pelvic Floor.* Beate Carriere and Dawn-Marie Ickes have written a book that shares consumer friendly descriptions of the basic anatomy and physiology of the pelvic floor and how to address a variety of conditions with pelvic floor exercises and physical therapy. Not only is this of great value to pelvic floor therapists, it gives us a better understanding of what is happening behind the doors of pelvic health programs. This gives clients and practitioners (both physicians and therapists) insight to the integration of pelvic floor fitness and physical therapy as an essential part of treating both men and women with pelvic floor issues.

Marc L. Winter, MD
Director of Benign Gynecology
Hoag Memorial Hospital Presbyterian
Member Hoag Memorial Hospital Presbyterian Center
of Excellence in Incontinence Care
Orange County, CA, USA

Preface

This book is dedicated to our colleagues who frequently ask for more treatment ideas. At the same time, it is dedicated to our patients to whom we are grateful for being our greatest teachers. We thank all patients who agreed to the videotaping of exercise sessions that demonstrate examples of faulty and correct breathing. The latter contributes to understanding the influence breathing has on the rehabilitation of the pelvic floor.

Thanks again to the colleagues Syndia Schafzahl, Johann Tengan, Joel Villamater, Georgine Hernandez, and Andrew Calasanz for their cooperation and help with the first edition of the book. Additional help for that project was also provided by Elsa Hodge, Jonathan, Max, and Lina Delbrück, Larisa and Nicola Salmon, Rachel De Perio, E. Guerrero, and R. Jones.

It is an honor to introduce Dawn-Marie Ickes, PT, MPT, PhD, PMA-CPT as co-author of the second edition. Dawn-Marie is Associate Professor in the Department of Physical Therapy at Mount Saint Mary's University in Los Angeles. In writing the second edition of *Fitness for the Pelvic Floor*, Dawn-Marie provided insight into what students and new therapists need to have in their toolbox for evaluation and exercise-based treatment interventions, while Beate provided new ideas for clinical applications.

Most of the cases presented in this book draw from experiences over Beate's five decades in practice.

We are grateful for the help and support we received from the people at Thieme in making the second edition of this book possible.

Beate Carrière, PT, CIFK, CAPP
Dawn-Marie Ickes, PT, MPT, PhD, PMA-CPT

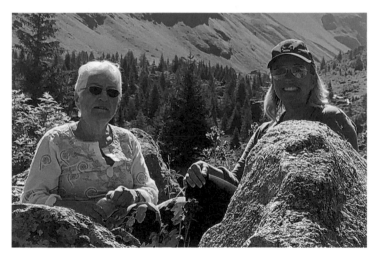

Beate Carrière　　　　　　　　Dawn-Marie Ickes

Introduction

Treatment Options and Exercises for Improving Physical and Sexual Health

Pelvic pain can manifest in a variety of ways in both men and women, ranging from symptoms of urgency to pain in the lower abdomen, vagina, rectum, perineum, and bony pelvis. The muscles that constitute the pelvic floor are often involved in pelvic pain, either as a driver of the problem or in response to the symptoms associated with the problem. Trauma to the pelvic girdle and its surrounding structures can result from gynecological procedures, abdominal or pelvic surgeries, infections, childbirth, sports-related injury, falling, poor posture for a sustained period of time, chronic straining due to constipation, and pelvic holding patterns related to stress.

Two hundred million people worldwide suffer from urinary incontinence.

Urinary incontinence is experienced by nearly 25 million individuals in the United States. It is estimated that the incidence of women with at least one pelvic floor disorder will nearly double from 28.1 million to 43.8 million by the year 2050.

Incontinence affects 1 in 3 women between the ages of 15 and 65 years, and between 1 and 3 out of 10 men within the same age range. Approximately 14% of adolescents under 15 years of age experience various forms of incontinence as well. In the US, incontinence-related costs exceeded $80 billion in 2020. The most common reason for admitting a family member to a nursing home is the family's inability to cope with incontinence.[1] Statistics show that between 50% and 65% of patients in nursing care facilities experience incontinence.[2] The idea that this is an issue one has to "just live with" is preposterous given that there are options available, many of which include strategies related to pelvic floor fitness. Most of us begin and end our lives in diapers.[3]

Although it is common to exercise many parts of the body to stay fit, very little attention is paid to exercising the pelvic floor. Perhaps we can prevent ending our lives in diapers if we devote some time exercising to keep the pelvic floor muscles fit.

Many exercises exist for the general fitness of the body, strengthening of the arms and legs, and the abdominal and back muscles. Finding fun exercises for the pelvic floor involves searching through a great deal of literature; finding exercises suitable for men, women, and children that are fun and effective appears to be impossible. It is also difficult to find exercises that can be done in therapy and at home with minimal cost. Additional options exist for treatment of the pelvic floor, but are mostly overlooked or not shared in a manner that is consumer friendly.

This book is designed to encourage patients to ask for help and provide therapists with creative treatment ideas, simple solutions for a wide range of pelvic floor related issues, and strategies for designing a program that respects the inherent variability of pelvic floor dysfunction while honoring the unique needs of each and every patient. The primary focus is on exercises; other treatment options are discussed but are not described in detail. The book is complemented by more than 50 videos.

An integrative approach is necessary where both the patient and therapist work together to solve the many mysteries connected to a pelvic floor that is not working properly. Some children or adults may suffer from bed-wetting at night, others do not dare to go out because of the sudden, irresistible urge of having to go to the bathroom when there is none nearby. Impairment of the pelvic floor in men and women of all ages causes leakage of urine when coughing, sneezing, or lifting objects. Others suffer from sexual problems such as pain or leakage of urine during intercourse and erectile dysfunctions. Some adults cannot control gas and feel impaired because they are embarrassed to be around other people. Many suffer from hemorrhoids and constipation, which may aggravate existing problems of the pelvic floor. A high number of silent sufferers are too embarrassed to seek help. It is time to speak up, see a doctor, and request a referral to see a therapist who can help restore pelvic floor function.

A hand-out sheet and squeezing exercises are no longer acceptable; the pelvic floor muscles deserve as much attention as, for example, a quadriceps muscle of the leg after a knee injury. In most cases the pelvic floor can be rehabilitated and its function restored. It all starts with understanding where you are currently and what is possible.

Our intention for this book is to increase the understanding of pelvic problems for anybody who is interested: patients, therapists, trainers, and caregivers alike. Often individuals who come for treatment are healthy but suffer from incontinence. Therefore, since the term "patient" is not always appropriate, "client" is also used; these terms are interchangeable.

It is very important for both the client/patient and the therapist to speak the same language and have a shared understanding of the invisible pelvic floor. Medical terms are thus used only when necessary and alternative descriptions to help guide the consumer are used. The reader will frequently see these terms placed in parentheses to allow the client/patient to familiarize themselves with the vocabulary. A glossary is included, which explains unfamiliar terms.

References

[1] Morrison A, Levy R. Fraction of nursing home admissions attributable to urinary incontinence. Value Health 2006;9 (4):272–274

[2] Bliss DZ, Harms S, Garrard JM, et al. Prevalence of incontinence by race and ethnicity of older people admitted to nursing homes. J Am Med Dir Assoc 2013;14(6):451.e1–451.e7

[3] Milsom I, Gyhagen M. The prevalence of urinary incontinence. Climacteric 2019;22(3):217–222

Navigating This Book

This book is divided into two parts and an appendix. The first part consists of a brief introduction to the anatomy and physiology of the pelvic floor and basic information about diaphragmatic breathing. Therapists will find more detailed information related to pathology, diagnostic testing, and etiology in textbooks. The reader can also learn about the purpose of keeping a bladder and bowel diary. This section explains the function of the pelvic floor muscles to patients with bladder and bowel incontinence specifically as this represents the fourth largest health-related expense for US citizens to date, with pneumonia, influenza, and breast cancer holding the first, second, and third rankings.

The second part of the book deals with exercises and treatment options. The appendices provide therapists with samples of evaluation forms for female and male patients with incontinence (Appendices A and B) and with forms that can be used before and after prostate surgery (Appendices C and D).

Part 1

**Anatomy and Physiology
of the Pelvic Floor**

1 Introduction

The pelvic floor is contained within the bony pelvis (▶ Fig. 1.1) and is made up of muscles, ligaments, nerves, fascia, and vascular structures that come together, creating a hammocklike support for the organs in the lowest part of the pelvis. It has four essential functions that are intimately related to one another. In addition to supporting the organs within the pelvis, it plays a role in bladder and bowel control, contributes to static and dynamic stabilization of the pelvic girdle, lumbar spine, and torso, and assists with sexual function.[24] The overlap in roles explains why muscular dysfunction in this area can cause a broad spectrum of challenges for men and women.

Pelvic floor muscular dysfunction (PFMD) refers to a wide range of disorders affecting one or, more commonly, a combination of the functions described. It occurs when the muscles are weak, tight, or torn, ligaments and/or fascia are stretched or damaged, resulting in an ineffective system for transferring loads through the pelvis. Often the direct causes are unknown; however, traumatic injuries, sexual abuse, strenuous exercise without proper breathing mechanics, and complications related to childbirth can contribute to the problem. The necessary support for the organs becomes imbalanced, affecting the normal functioning of the lower intestines, bowel, bladder, uterus, vagina, and rectum.

A careful evaluation prior to treatment may indicate which systems are involved. Sometimes the dysfunction can be very complicated and warrants a thorough investigation by a knowledgeable physical therapist and a physician. An experienced therapist may, in addition to training the fast and slow muscle fibers, select other treatment options (e.g., breathing exercises, manual therapy, connective tissue manipulation, soft-tissue mobilization, biofeedback, electrical stimulation, and heat or cold application). Understanding the complexity of possible involvement is especially important when treating patients with pelvic floor pain.[67] A one-size-fits-all approach to addressing PFMD simply will not work. Taking a biographical approach to obtaining a client's history can help tell the story that lies within the tissues and informs what is necessary to help the client in a meaningful way. Consideration of the client's individuality and sensitivity to challenges which may be related to emotional and physical abuse are essential to creating a nonthreatening environment where one can heal. The effects of trauma can impact the survivor's experience of the entire process of care, health-related behaviors, and outcomes.[60] Establishing rapport, detailing the process, expectations, and placing the client in a position of comfort while being mindful of language use are essential. Being aware not to sit higher than the client during the intake can make a world of difference.

The muscles of the pelvic floor have the same capabilities as any other muscle in the body; they

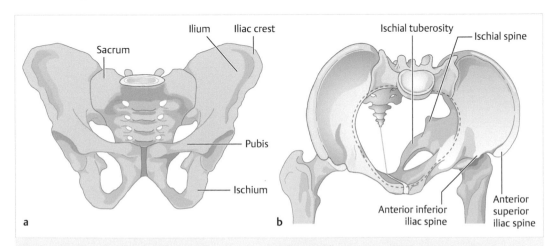

Fig. 1.1 (a) The bony pelvis. (b) The dashed line (– – –) indicates the plane of the pelvic inlet; the solid line (——) indicates the plane of the pelvic outlet. Reproduced from Carrière B, Feldt CM. The Pelvic Floor. 1st Edition. Stuttgart: Thieme; 2006.

must be able to contract, relax, elongate, and give feedback. If one cannot effectively contract the muscles, they may experience inadequate support for the organs, pelvic girdle, urethra, or sphincter. Difficulty with relaxing the muscles can result in lower back pain, pain during intercourse, inability to completely empty the bladder, and painful trigger points within the muscles of the pelvic girdle. The inability to elongate the muscles can also result in constipation and digestive issues.

The debilitating impact of urinary incontinence (UI) represents a condition in young people that has the most substantial negative impact on "health-related quality of life" (▶ Fig. 1.1). In older individuals, next to stroke and Alzheimer's disease, UI is reported to have the most negative effect on "health-related quality of life."[59,62] The cost of incontinence-related care is astonishing. This fact, combined with the 6.5-year average length of time from when individuals first experience bladder control symptoms to when they seek medical attention, is our call to action. The time has come to address the issue through education, conversation, and a specialized approach to designing pelvic floor fitness programs.

1.1 Basic Bladder Neurophysiology

Various micturition (voiding) centers in the brain and spinal cord are involved in emptying the bladder. These centers control the reflexes to empty the bladder and coordinate its filling. Some of the reflexes involved in this process can be inhibited by voluntary control. In the bladder emptying phase, a signal from these nerves coordinates the detrusor contraction and urethral sphincter relaxation. The voluntary relaxation of the urethral sphincter and pelvic floor while the detrusor muscle contracts and empties the bladder (▶ Fig. 1.2).

A unique feature of the bladder is that emptying (voiding) can be delayed or done early, even when the bladder is not full. A person usually empties the bladder when it is most convenient, typically every 2 to 4 hours during the daytime and less at night.

An important micturition center lies in the brainstem. Information from the bladder first reaches the micturition center of the sacral spine before being relayed to the brainstem. The micturition center of the brainstem conveys the information that the bladder is filling up to the brain (cortex). It also relays messages to other essential areas within the brain, such as the limbic system (center for motivation and memory) and the cerebellum (responsible for muscle control). The connection to the cortex enables a person to make a conscious decision to delay micturition or to empty the bladder early.

Therefore, patients who suffer from a stroke or Alzheimer's disease, which can result in damage to some regions of the brain, can experience problems. They may not remember that they can postpone emptying the bladder, or they may be unmotivated, depending on the injury to the brain. It is also possible that the cerebellum is damaged and that the muscles cannot be well adjusted and therefore do not function optimally.

With poor memory, it may be necessary to prompt voiding by reminding the patient to empty the bladder regularly. With other patients, timed voiding may be required, which means that the patient is placed at regular intervals on a toilet to empty the bowel or bladder. With timed voiding, some patients afflicted with dementia can stay dry.

Patients with spinal cord injuries often suffer from damage to the tracts connecting the micturition center in the sacral region with that in the brainstem. These patients are no longer able to influence voiding voluntarily. The use of a catheter may be required. Tapping the bladder or other tricks (such as a brief manual stretch of the external anal sphincter muscle) can trigger bladder emptying by eliciting relaxation of the pelvic floor muscles. Relaxation is a prerequisite for the contraction of the bladder muscle. If it works, the short reflex arc from the bladder to the sacral micturition center and back to the bladder causes the bladder to empty.

Bladder infections may cause the short arc reflex to be overactive, resulting in a great desire to empty the bladder, called an "urgency." If the reflex activity is not functioning correctly, it can also cause a "spasm" of the bladder muscle, resulting in a strong urge to empty the bladder immediately. It is most important not to move when this happens; in fact, it helps to try to actively relax the muscles with deep breathing and a conscious effort to relax. It may also be beneficial to perform a few quick contractions of the pelvic floor muscles ("quick flicks"), as this may contribute to normalizing the irregular reflex activity. Distraction can help in some cases. With practice, such contractions can help to delay emptying consciously and to overcome the urgency.

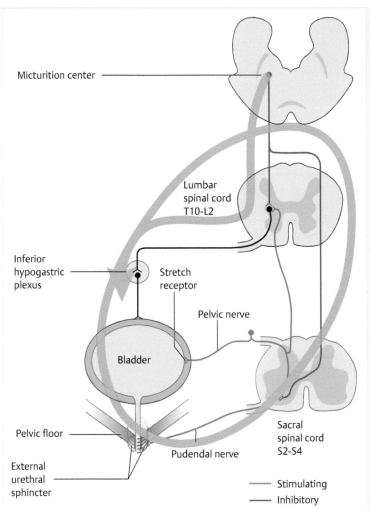

Fig. 1.2 Viscerosomatic loop. Modified from Carrière B, Feldt CM. The Pelvic Floor 1st Edition. Stuttgart: Thieme; 2006.

Micturition center

Lumbar spinal cord T10-L2

Inferior hypogastric plexus

Stretch receptor

Pelvic nerve

Bladder

Pelvic floor

External urethral sphincter

Pudendal nerve

Sacral spinal cord S2-S4

—— Stimulating

—— Inhibitory

Finally, strong pelvic floor muscles provide a solid base for the bladder and can be instrumental in overcoming urge incontinence. Because the external sphincter muscles are part of the skeletal pelvic floor muscles, their strength may help to control urgencies.

The pelvic floor muscles are innervated by the pudendal nerve, which originates in sacral roots 2 to 4 of the spinal cord. The nerve reacts to information from the micturition centers. Injury to the pudendal nerve (such as stretching during a difficult birth or damage sustained through a fall on the sacrum) prevents the pelvic floor muscles from contracting correctly. The muscle tonus may be too low and the muscles weak. This can result in urinary or anal incontinence, inability to control gas, or dysfunction of the pelvic floor muscles, even if all reflexes are intact. Interestingly, the pelvic floor muscles have a higher resting tone than other skeletal muscles. This is to ensure continence at night.

Various reflexes (some of which are not yet fully understood) are finely coordinated with the activity of the pelvic floor muscles. It is believed that the transverse abdominal muscle influences the strength of the pelvic floor and assists in providing continence.[58]

The autonomic nervous system (▶ Fig. 1.3) is connected in the sacral area (parasympathetic nerve fibers) and upper lumbar region (sympathetic nerve fibers) with the spinal cord and helps regulate all the reflexes. The autonomic nervous system coordinates the function of the inner organs with the function of the organs supported

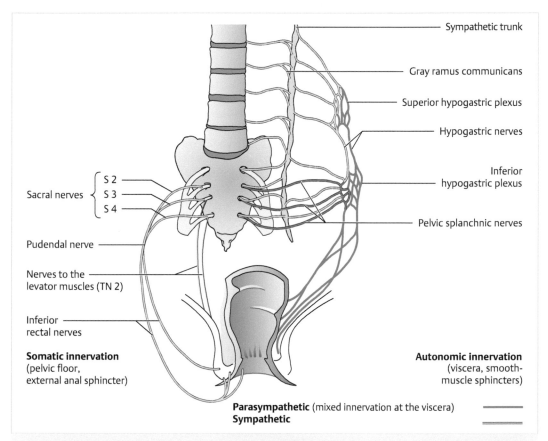

Fig. 1.3 The autonomic nervous system (according to Hirschfeld and Léveillé). Reproduced from Carrière B, Feldt CM. The Pelvic Floor. 1st Edition. Stuttgart: Thieme; 2006.

by the pelvic floor via the viscerosomatic loop (See also ▶ Fig. 1.2). Fear or anxiety originating in the brain can, therefore, cause diarrhea, inability to void, nausea, cold sweaty hands, increased heart rate, etc. Injuries to the nerves of the autonomic nervous system usually cause diffuse pain. Breathing exercises can help calm down an autonomic system in distress.

Pearl

When a person cannot sit without severe pain in the pelvic floor, but has no pain while standing or lying in a horizontal position, then it is likely that the pudendal nerve is the cause and needs attention.

2 Layers of the Pelvic Floor

The pelvic girdle is a deep and somewhat narrow region of the lower torso which houses intestinal, urologic and gynaecologic viscera, nerves, muscles, vessels and fascial connections. By design, it works to adequately suspend the structures it contains and promote synchronized function during elimination. Multi-compartmental dysfunction can arise from damage to the functional or structural relationships within the pelvis.

The pelvic floor can be viewed in three layers functioning as a dome-shaped complex with muscles contracting in the sagittal, frontal, and transverse planes. Sometimes the third layer is described as two different layers because the deep transverse perineal muscle lies deeper than the other muscles of the urogenital diaphragm.

2.1 First Layer—Parietalis Fascia (Formerly Endopelvic Fascia)

The first layer is called the parietalis fascia, formerly known as the endopelvic fascia (▶ Fig. 2.1). It functions as a suspensory apparatus for the pelvic organs. It is a lining that covers the pelvic walls formed by a complex of smooth muscle fibers, ligaments, nerves, blood vessels, and connective tissue; it supports and covers the bladder, the inner organs such as the intestine, rectum, and the uterus in women and the prostate in men, thus connecting the interior of the pelvis to the lower extremity.

Within this layer are three critical relationships of loose fiber-rich connective tissue and fascia, surrounded by blood vessels, nerves and lymphatic structures that sling the pelvic viscera from the walls of the pelvis. These include the cardinal ligaments, uterosacral ligaments, and the pubocervical ligaments. These three ligaments serve as support to the vault of the vagina and the cervix in women.

The loose connective tissue surrounding the pelvic organs serves to adapt to the dynamic changes of these organs and their interfaces, which are functionally variable.

Some of the ligaments of the parietalis fascia connect to the lumbar spine and the symphysis pubis. Even though this layer cannot be exercised, training the pelvic floor muscles of the second layer (pelvic diaphragm) can improve back pain by increasing the support of the bladder and uterus from below and decreasing the strain on the ligaments upon which the support otherwise depends. Strong pelvic floor muscles can help support the bladder, uterus, and rectum if a person has sustained tears of the parietalis fascia through childbirth or other injury.

2.2 Second Layer (Pelvic Diaphragm)

The levator ani, "the lifter of the anus," is the most crucial muscle forming the pelvic floor (▶ Fig. 2.2). It is a muscle group that spans between the sitting

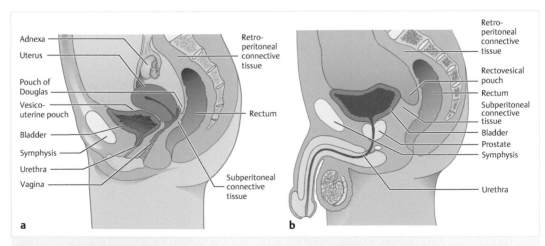

Fig. 2.1 First layer of the pelvic floor (parietal/endopelvic fascia; side view). **(a)** Female. **(b)** Male. Reproduced from Carrière B, Feldt CM. The Pelvic Floor. 1st Edition. Stuttgart: Thieme; 2006.

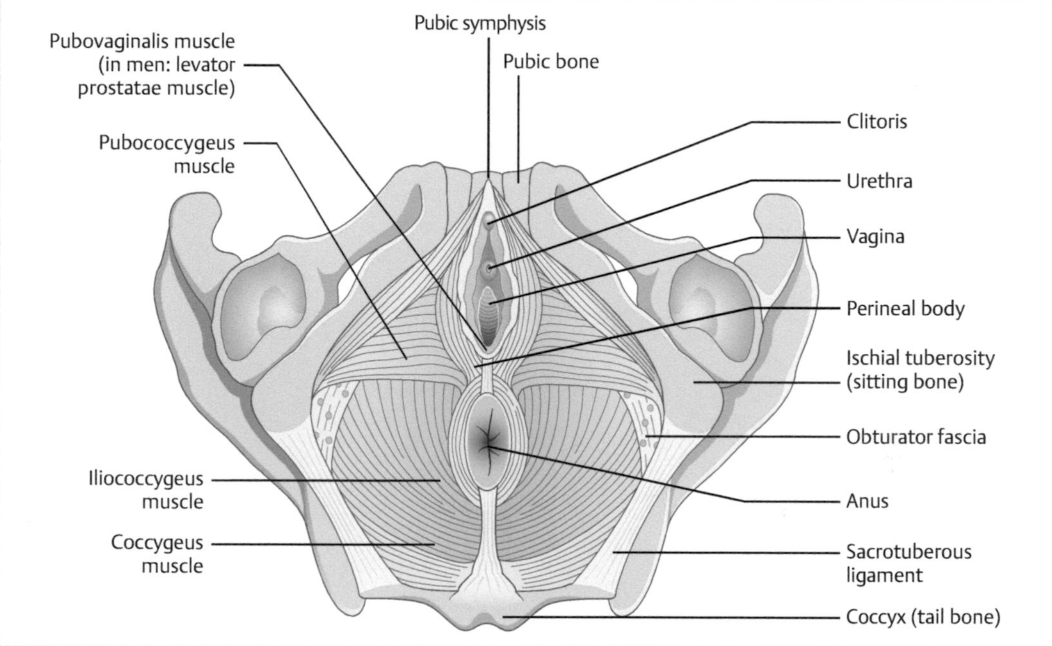

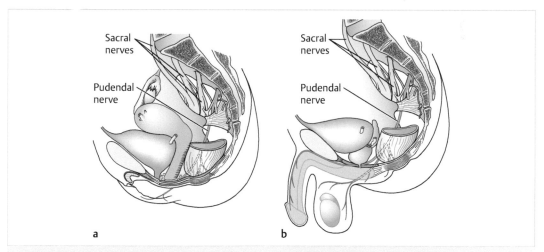

Fig. 2.2 Second layer of the pelvic floor (pelvic diaphragm; levator ani muscle; view from below, the urogenital diaphragm is not visible in this view). Reproduced from Carrière B, Feldt CM. The Pelvic Floor. 1st Edition. Stuttgart: Thieme; 2006.

Fig. 2.3 The pudendal nerve and sacral nerves. **(a)** Female. **(b)** Male. Reproduced from Carrière B, Feldt CM. The Pelvic Floor.1st Edition. Stuttgart: Thieme; 2006.

bones and between the tail bone (coccyx) and pubic bones. The levator ani muscle provides support for all the organs of the pelvis and guarantees continence at night. Therefore, it differs from other skeletal muscles in that it is has a high resting tone naturally. The pudendal nerve innervates it.

The pudendal nerve innervates all of the above muscles of the pelvic diaphragm and urogenital diaphragm. Because this nerve also has sensory fibers, it can contribute to perineal (area between anus and vagina) and pelvic pain. Blood vessels (arteries) deliver oxygen to the muscles of the pelvic floor (▶ Fig. 2.3).

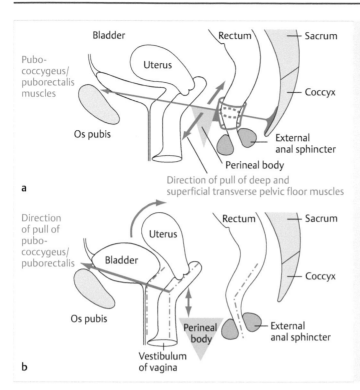

Fig. 2.4 Support of the uterus by the perineal body. (a) Empty bladder. (b) Full bladder. Reproduced from Carrière B, Feldt CM. The Pelvic Floor. 1st Edition. Stuttgart: Thieme; 2006.

When coughing and sneezing, quick precontractions are required to maintain continence (▶ Fig. 2.4).

In response to these needs, the muscles have approximately 70% slow-twitch muscle fibers and 30% fast-twitch muscle fibers.[54] The slow fiber (type 1-aerobic) and fast fiber (type 2-anaerobic) types provide both strength endurance and balance energy consumption for pelvic floor muscle function. The fast-twitch, which generates energy anaerobically, provides a quick and powerful contraction with 20% more force compared to the slow-twitch fibers.

The levator ani has several parts fanning out in different directions (▶ Fig. 2.5):
- *The pubococcygeus muscle.* Its fibers extend from the pubic bones to the tail bone. A contraction sometimes can be felt at the side of the tip of the tail bone.
- *The puborectalis muscle.* Fibers of this critical muscle loop around the rectum, pulling it forward during contraction and assisting with providing continence.
- *The iliococcygeus muscle* extends from the tail bone to each of the sitting bones. Some of

these muscle fibers run from one side to the other, some in a more diagonal direction.

Additional muscles which work synergistically with the levator ani at this level:
- *The pubovaginalis muscle* (in women only) loops around the vagina. These fibers run in the front to back direction.
- *The levator prostatae muscle* (in men only) supports the prostate gland.
- *The coccygeus muscle* lies adjacent to the iliococcygeus muscle. It can influence the stability of the sacroiliac joint. Abnormal tension of the muscle can keep the sacroiliac joint in a displaced position.[63]
- *The internal sphincter muscles* of the bladder and the rectum consist of smooth muscle fibers and cannot be trained with active exercises. Especially during radical surgery of the prostate, the internal sphincter of the bladder can be removed or damaged. Therefore, patients depend on the function of the skeletal muscles of the pelvic floor to stay dry.

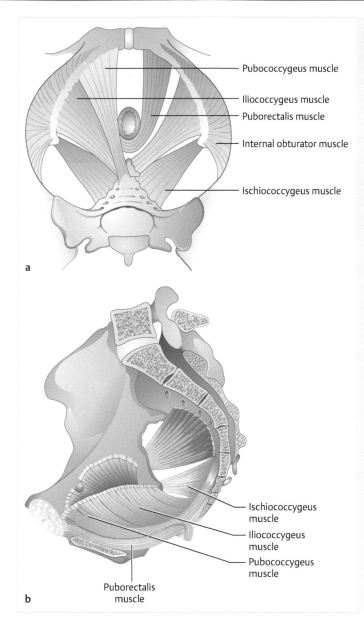

Pubococcygeus muscle

Iliococcygeus muscle

Puborectalis muscle

Internal obturator muscle

Ischiococcygeus muscle

a

Ischiococcygeus muscle

Iliococcygeus muscle

Pubococcygeus muscle

Puborectalis muscle

b

Fig. 2.5 (a, b) The muscles of the pelvic floor. Reproduced from Carrière B, Feldt CM. The Pelvic Floor. 1st Edition. Stuttgart: Thieme; 2006.

2.3 Third Layer (Urogenital Diaphragm)

The outer layer of the pelvic floor consists of several muscles. The deep transverse perineal muscle is vital for continence and supports the function of the levator ani. The other muscles of this layer are essential for sexual purposes. The muscles of the third layer do not support the organs of the pelvis (▶ Fig. 2.6).

- *The deep transverse perineal muscle* provides additional fibers, such as the sphincter urethra loops around the urethra in men and women, and assists with continence. It is under voluntary control. The muscle fibers run from side to side.

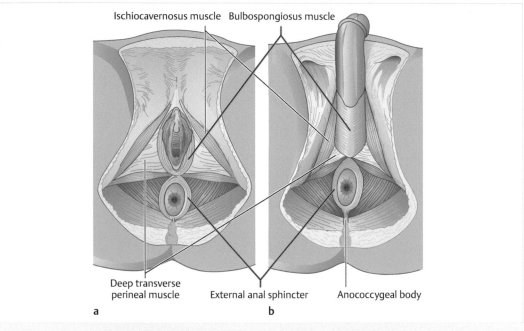

Fig. 2.6 The muscles external to the pelvic floor. **(a)** Female. **(b)** Male. Reproduced from Carrière B, Feldt CM. The Pelvic Floor. 1st Edition. Stuttgart: Thieme; 2006.

- *The superficial transverse perineal muscle* reinforces the action of the deep transverse perineus. The muscle fibers also run from side to side.
- *The bulbocavernosus muscle (musculus bulbospongiosus)* connects (in men) the bulb of the penis to the urogenital diaphragm and contracts during ejaculation and at the end of urination. In women, it contracts during orgasm,
erecting the clitoris. The muscle fibers run in a front to back direction.
- *The ischiocavernous muscle* has an essential function in men since it assists in increasing the erection. The muscle fibers run in a diagonal direction. In women, it erects the clitoris.
- *The anal sphincter muscle* loops around the anus like a ring and provides continence of the rectum.

3 Evaluation of Breathing

Evaluation and restoration of abdominal breathing is required to ensure coordination of the function of the entire abdominal compartment for all clients with *any* form of pelvic floor muscular dysfunction (PFMD) (▶ Fig. 3.1 and ▶ Fig. 3.3). Therapists' keen observational and listening skills are essential to identifying the extent of the breathing dysfunction affecting the pelvic floor muscles and internal pelvic organs.

Normal breathing: The pulmonary diaphragm moves downward during inhalation, the abdomen widens, and the pelvic floor moves slightly downward if it is resilient and relaxed (▶ Fig. 3.2). The abdomen responds to exhalation, flattens, and then the pulmonary diaphragm moves again

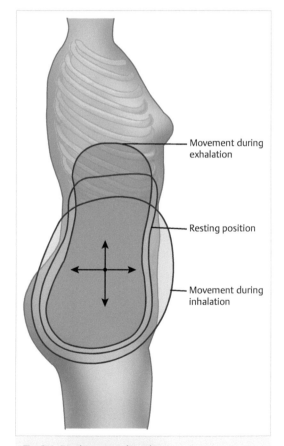

Fig. 3.1 Diaphragmatic breathing.

Movement during exhalation

Resting position

Movement during inhalation

upward with only minimal upward movement of the chest. Resting one hand on the chest (to feel minimal movement on the chest) and the other just below the rib cage, the abdominal movement below the rib cage flaring outward can be felt with inhaling and flaring gently inward during exhalation. When looking at the upper torso, the clavicles (collar bones) are positioned in an oblique direction from the sternum upward and backward (▶ Fig. 3.3, ▶ Video 3.1). This oblique alignment is necessary for normal breathing.

Faulty breathing is observed in standing or sitting as well as lying on the back. Clients who primarily breathe with the upper torso may have their clavicles in a horizontal position and the muscles of the neck may assist to pull the chest upward (▶ Fig. 3.3). The neck muscles can be very tight, and the neck may not look relaxed. The epigastric angle could be very wide, more than 90 degrees. Even with clothes on, there could be a deep crease visible above the navel (▶ Video 3.3). When lying on the back, the crease can be three to four fingers deep, which made me call it the "Grand Canyon" of the abdomen (▶ Video 3.4). Usually, the transverse abdominal muscle and the oblique abdominal muscles are very weak. Tight upper neck muscles and weak trunk muscles are expected. The client may also have a poor posture in need of restoration (▶ Video 3.6).

With the client sitting or lying on the back, one can observe and palpate how the breathing movement is only going toward the neck from the crease above the navel. Their breath may not be expanding to the pelvic diaphragm, reaching the pelvic floor. The lungs do not expand downward. I tell my clients that the lungs and heart movements are restricted (in jail and need to be liberated). It may take several treatments to correct such breathing. The clients tell me that they feel liberated when the lungs and heart can move more freely, and the neck muscles are relaxed (▶ Video 3.1 and ▶ Video 3.2). Scar tissue in the area between the anus and vagina can make the pelvic floor tissue less pliable and cause a hypertonicity, preventing downward mobility of the pelvic floor.

Reversed breathing: It is not uncommon to see clients suck the air upward and pull the belly

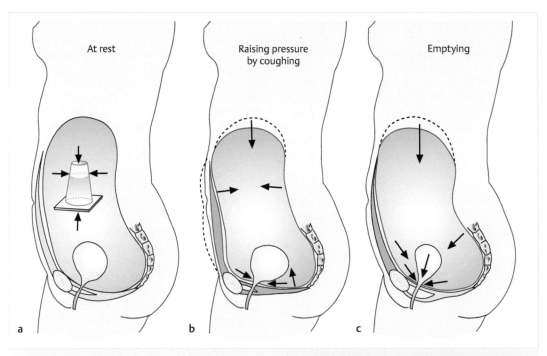

Fig. 3.2 (a–c) Interaction of the pulmonary diaphragm and the pelvic floor muscles. Reproduced from Carrière B, Feldt CM. The Pelvic Floor. 1st Edition. Stuttgart: Thieme; 2006.

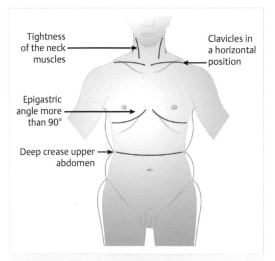

Fig. 3.3 Typical signs of breathing dysfunction (marked with red lines).

Tightness of the neck muscles

Clavicles in a horizontal position

Epigastric angle more than 90°

Deep crease upper abdomen

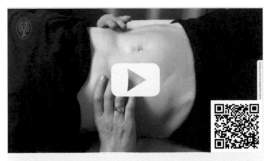

Video 3.1 Breath assessment demonstrating correct widening of the lower ribs

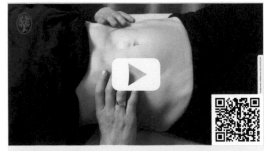

Video 3.2 Corrected diaphragmatic breathing with lower rib widening and minimal chest movement

inward while pushing on the pelvic floor during exhalation(▶ Video 3.8). It is not a good idea when organs within the pelvis are pushed downward (▶ Video 3.5). One of my clients was sent with a diagnosis of a prolapse (too long intestine)

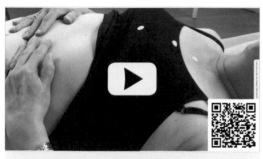

Video 3.3 Example of faulty breathing

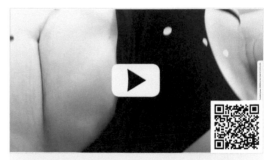

Video 3.4 Faulty upper torso breathing with deep crease above navel (also known as "Grand Canyon" pattern)

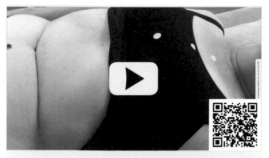

Video 3.5 Faulty breathing with abnormal chest movement and hollowing of pelvis

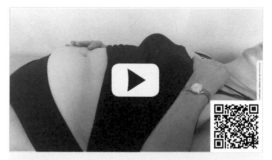

Video 3.6 Corrected "Grand Canyon" pattern

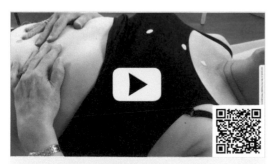

Video 3.7 Faulty breathing-chest

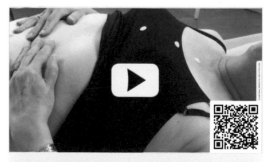

Video 3.8 Reverse faulty breathing with sucking in of air and pushing belly out with exhalation

and scheduled for surgery (▶ Video 3.10). Careful observation solved the problem. At the end of diaphragmatic breathing, the client sucked the belly, like a wave, inward and backward, pushing forcefully onto the colon. When the client learned not to press downward and to exhale with the awareness of relaxation, her colon shortened again, and she did not require surgery.

Reversed panting: Just like reversed breathing, clients suck the air in and push down into the pelvic floor facilitating prolapse of inner organs of the pelvis (▶ Video 3.9).

Pearl

Observation of breathing from the beginning to the end. This assessment is best when the abdomen is not covered with clothing. It is of utmost importance to restore the health of the client, not only for the pelvic floor but also for the heart and lungs and to prevent prolapse of inner organs. Trunk muscles need to be strengthened, the mobility of the ribs and the pelvic floor restored, and the breathing patterns corrected (▶ Video 3.3, ▶ Video 3.4, ▶ Video 3.5, and ▶ Video 3.7).

3.1 Treatment of Breathing Dysfunction

Poor breathing patterns are so common that correct breathing (together with proper lifting) should be taught in kindergarten. The command "pull your stomach in" may be a cause of faulty breathing patterns and "chest breathing" for many who were told this in years past. A shift in fashions and ideals is another contributing factor. Some men tend to pull in their stomachs because it makes their chest appear more substantial. Patterns of movement, positioning, and breathing are now seen as potential sources for musculoskeletal dysfunction; for example, back problems due to the lumbar spine losing its flexibility and the center of gravity changing with a raised chest.

The neck muscles can become tight because they cannot relax when used for breathing. Breathing primarily with the chest also prevents the pelvic floor muscles from working in union (synergy) with the pulmonary diaphragm (▶ Fig. 3.2).

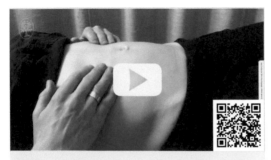

Video 3.9 Panting technique demonstrating abdomen rising and pushing out followed by panting correction (note chest is quiet with proper panting)

3.2 Correction of Breathing Patterns

It is essential to correct faulty breathing patterns, not only for the sake of the pelvic floor muscles but also to decrease strain on the neck muscles. Proper breathing may improve the oxygen supply to the pelvic floor through its many arteries (see ▶ Fig. 2.3). Oxygen is a requirement for well-functioning muscles. Abdominal breathing coordinates the pulmonary diaphragm with the pelvic diaphragm and helps to promote healthy bowel movements by maintaining the proper balance of internal pressure in this region. The abdominal and back muscles train optimally when breathing coordinates correctly during activities such as walking, running, and lifting. The risk of back injuries is reduced by a well-trained torso, a well-aligned body, and balanced flexibility supporting good posture (see Chapter 12 [p. 47]).

Breathing can be practiced sitting, standing, kneeling, or lying on the side, stomach, or back (▶ Video 3.6, ▶ Video 3.10, ▶ Video 3.11, ▶ Video 3.12, ▶ Video 3.13, and ▶ Video 3.14).

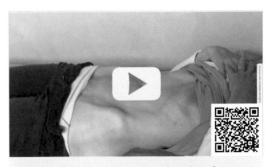

Video 3.10 Example of corrective breathing for a lengthened colon

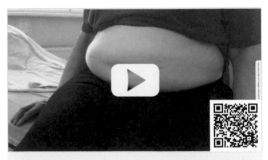

Video 3.11 Corrected breathing in sitting position

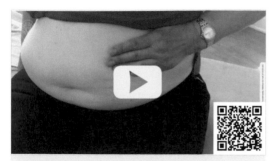

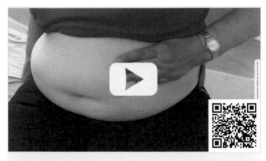

Video 3.12 Corrected breathing in sitting position with use of hand

Video 3.13 Upright sitting correction with use of hand to cue obliques

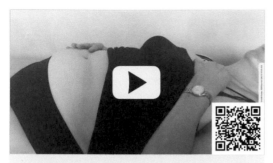

Video 3.14 Self-awareness and corrective breathing and panting in supine position with two hands

3.3 Observation of the Shape of the Rib Cage

Evaluating posture and the shape of the chest, rib cage, and abdomen may provide insight into potential respiratory problems.

- If the angle formed by the rib cage is greater than 90 degrees, this may indicate a breathing dysfunction, possibly secondary to weak oblique abdominal muscles and reduced downward movement of the pulmonary diaphragm.

- Horizontally positioned collar bones can indicate a possible postural and breathing problem. The scalene muscles may be tight (see ▶ Fig. 3.3). A therapist can further evaluate which corrective exercises may be necessary.
- Does the abdomen rise during inhalation and fall during exhalation?
- Does the movement come primarily from the chest or the belly?
- In normal breathing, the abdomen rises and then the rib cage expands; the sternum lifts only slightly (see ▶ Fig. 9.1 and ▶ Fig. 9.2).
- Breathing primarily with the chest is a common faulty breathing pattern.
- Another incorrect breathing pattern is to reverse the breathing, sucking the stomach in during inhalation and pushing it out during exhalation.
- Equally erroneous is the correct rising of the abdomen during inhalation and flattening of the abdomen during exhalation but with "pouching" of the lower abdomen at the end of exhalation, usually with an increase of abdominal pressure.

4 Functions of the Pelvic Floor Muscles

It is essential to understand the many roles of the pelvic floor. Of equal importance is understanding what kind of dysfunctions can be caused by a weak (low-tone dysfunction, LTD) versus a stiff (high-tone dysfunction, HTD) pelvic floor. Strength does not always equate with optimal function. Nearly 68% of women experience one or more problems associated with pelvic floor dysfunction (PFD), organ prolapse, or incontinence.[51] Injuries, deterioration of muscles, nerve, ligaments and facial, which support and maintain the infrastructure for optimal pelvic function, can lead to debilitating pelvic floor dysfunction, such as organ prolapse and incontinence.

4.1 Bladder and Bowel Function —Elimination and Continence

The pelvic floor muscles must be strong enough to support the bladder, vagina, rectum, and the inner organs of the abdomen. Relaxation of the muscles is required when expelling feces and urine and when giving birth. The muscles provide continence when lifting heavy objects and when sleeping. During coughing, sneezing, running, and jumping, quick contractions prevent leakage of urine.

4.2 Pelvic Girdle Stability

Instability of the pelvic girdle can result in musculoskeletal issues of the sacroiliac joints, lumbar spine, and hips locally, not to mention the global more peripheral effects that clients experience. Pudendal nerve entrapment, obturator internus syndrome, and piriformis syndrome are common diagnoses associated with deficits in pelvic girdle stability.

The pelvic floor muscles work together (in synergy) with the dome-shaped breathing muscle, the pulmonary diaphragm, which sits behind the sternum. Its primary purpose is to regulate the pressure between the thorax and the abdomen. All abdominal muscles contribute to respiration.[47,48]

The abdominal, back, and hip muscles have to coordinate with the activity of the pelvic floor muscles.[65]

4.3 Sexual Function—Arousal and Pleasure

During sexual activities and orgasm, the pelvic floor muscles contract voluntarily or even involuntarily. Clients who have been sexually abused often have a high tone in their pelvic floor muscles. Occasionally this can lead to an overflow bladder (constant dripping of urine). Breathing dysfunction is also common. One client pushed downward onto the pelvic floor during exhalation, as a defense mechanism, causing colon problems. It is essential to listen carefully to the clients during history taking and assure them that no internal treatment will occur unless both the client and the therapist agreed that it would be necessary. Make sure you are not sitting higher—not looking down to a client who may be an abuse survivor. In addition, positioning yourself at eye level or below helps to ensure that you are not assuming a subconsciously dominant position.

Case Example

A 14-year-old young client was constantly dripping urine for 2 years and was in great despair; she was called diaper-girl in school and could not participate in sport and had to leave school because of the shame. All kinds of treatments by various doctors did not help. When I asked her doctor if she had a history of abuse, he said that 2 years ago, an aggressor was unable to penetrate her pelvic floor, because the girl tightened her legs so tight. At this moment, it was clear to me that the girl had to learn to relax her high-tone pelvic floor, restore the sensory awareness of the trunk, pelvis, and legs, and also understand the function of the bladder. After 10 treatments, this cooperative, intelligent girl was able to urinate properly, and her health was restored. In another school, she was one of the best students in her class.

With all clients who have experienced sexual abuse, it is crucial to understand that they may have difficulty saying no, because "no" in the past did not help. A hesitant yes and lack of eye contact may be a "no" in reality. Take time to allow the client to process the questions you are asking them.

5 Understanding Tone Differences in the Pelvic Floor Muscles

Pelvic floor dysfunction (PFD) relates to impairments in tone, muscle recruitment timing and patterns, and contractile force within the muscles that constitute the pelvic floor. As variable and unique as the individuals experiencing PFD, the dysfunctions are categorized as low tone or high tone to help differentiate the types of exercise-based treatment options that exist.[44]

Training the entire abdominal compartment is essential when restoring an imbalanced (either weak, hypotonic, or excessively tight/stiff or hypertonic) pelvic floor. Once the muscle can work in many combinations, it will most likely continue to train itself automatically during daily activities. An example of this is how the four muscles (quadriceps) that make up leg would work after rehabilitation. There are many options to choose from, allowing the brain to recruit the muscle activities it needs for the specific action desired.

5.1 Pelvic Floor Weakness (Low-Tone Dysfunction)

This condition is characterized as low-tone dysfunction (LTD). Muscles with this diagnosis are typically thin and atrophied with laxity of the anal sphincter and a broader vaginal vault (the space where one would place a tampon). Pain with palpation is not usually an issue. Volitional control is difficult for the client. Contractions are described as weak and diminish with endurance, not within the functional norm of 10 quick contractions and a 10-second hold with sustained contractions.[29,44] LTD is more common in nulliparous women and may involve denervation from stretching of the pudendal nerve and generalized connective tissue laxity.

The most common example is stress incontinence, which is caused by weakness of the pelvic floor and can associate with urgencies during the day. In men, weakness of the pelvic floor is more common after prostate surgery. The combination of urgency, with or without loss of urine, and frequent urination during the day and also at night (nocturia) is called overactive bladder (OAB). Women who suffer from loss of urine during activities of daily living (ADL), namely, lifting children, carrying groceries, and frequent bending, commonly suffer from LTD. Pelvic floor muscle (PFM) exercises guide the restoration of muscle function and assist in diminishing the symptoms of LTD symptoms of incontinence, urgency, and frequency.[29]

5.1.1 Consequences of Weak (Low-Tone) Pelvic Floor Muscles

The consequences of weak PFMs can be devastating. The lives of many women and men become restricted due, for example, to:
- Embarrassment because of leaking urine when coughing or sneezing
- Frequent runs to the bathroom and not wanting to go anywhere because of a fear of not finding a toilet in time
- Broken bones (fractures) secondary to falls when rushing to the bathroom, or unable to remove clothes quickly
- Fear of leakage of urine when performing exercise, such as aerobics, gym exercises, walking, and running
- Sitting on a warm surface—a reaction of afferent input to the cerebellum in the brain to relax the PFMs
- Fear of laughing (called giggle incontinence, affecting mostly teenagers), resulting in not going out with friends because of fear of losing urine when laughing
- Fear that others may smell the leaked urine, resulting in social isolation
- Sexual problems, possibly secondary to prolapse of the uterus, vagina, rectum, or bladder, an inability to contract the muscles tightly, and possible loss of urine during sexual intercourse
- Incontinence, possibly causing depression and sleep deprivation

Case Example

One time, I had a client who did not suffer from loss of urine, but she had a tremendous fear that she possibly could suffer from loss of urine on a planned trip to Russia. During the history taking, it turned out that the client grew up in the Netherlands and was in hiding in an attic during the occupation, always fearing of losing urine.

The "treatment" was to explain the function of the bladder and how much it could hold. Fast and slow muscle training was reviewed. When the client told me that she was going on a weekend vacation place in California, I encouraged her to hike in the mountains where she did not know where the next bathroom would be (in an emergency, there would always be a tree).

The client found out that she was able to go for a long hike without having to urinate, and that gave her the confidence to have no problems during her upcoming travel. She was also encouraged to wear a pad for just in case she was unable to find a bathroom. The client reported that she did well in Russia with no fear of loss of urine.

Pearl

Weak muscles cause leakage of urine/bowel. Tight PFMs cause the inability to relax the muscle, and urination often is not spontaneous, hesitant, and often painful. Anismus is a term for a very tight sphincter muscle of the anus. Vaginismus is the tightness of the vagina and can cause pain with even desired penetration during intercourse. Relaxation education and focused breathing can help to relax, gently stretching of the muscles can help (▶ Video 5.3), and also tools (e.g., cones) can help. A trained therapist can instruct and advise how to treat LTD.

5.2 Pelvic Floor Stiffness or "Short" Pelvic Floor Muscles (High-Tone Dysfunction)

Pelvic floor trauma, chronic strain, mechanical dysfunction, as a result of poor breathing mechanics, or incorrect training patterns can result from excessive force and/or overuse. Muscles with this diagnosis may feel boggy, thickened with hypertrophic and taut bands within the muscles. Palpation is painful and often difficult to access. Contractions may be weak and endurance limited (similar to high-tone dysfunction [HTD] but via a different mechanism).

Symptoms include voiding frequency, stress incontinence, pelvic pain, dyspareunia, and urgency.[74] The tight and inflexible pelvic floor may be durable, but the inability to lengthen and relax the muscles creates relative stiffness. Trigger points within the muscle itself are frequently present, and this condition is characterized as HTD. Clients can have urgencies or frequently try to urinate, but have difficulty to start urination, also described as hesitance. Exercises that gently stretch the tight muscles can improve the flexibility of the PFMs

Approximately 25 million Americans suffer from bladder or bowel problems, yet an estimated one-third of those affected do not discuss the issue with their doctor because it is too embarrassing.[21,51] Many individuals with urine or bowel incontinence suffer in silence. Very seldom doctors ask patients about bladder and bowel problems, feeling equally at odds to discuss this matter. One study found that nearly two-thirds of women with urinary incontinence have not discussed their symptoms with their health care provider.[41]

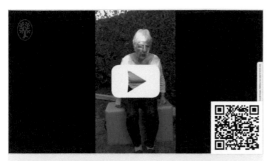

Video 5.1 Seated skill and coordination exercises

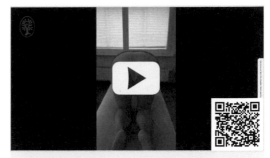

Video 5.2 Pelvic floor stretch in quadruped position

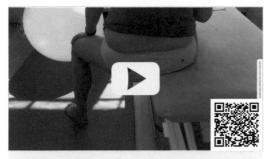

Video 5.3 Pelvic floor stretch in sitting position

(▶ Video 5.1) or increase the distance between the tight muscles between the sitting bone (▶ Video 5.2).

PFMs that are chronically tight pull and strain their relationships with other structures, including muscles, ligaments, bones, and fascia. This elevated tone results in an imbalance (usually increase) of pressure on neighboring structures such as the bladder, prostate, and rectum, impacting proper function and blood flow.

Other consequences of a stiff, nonrelaxing, short or stiff pelvic floor include pain with vaginal penetration, building arousal, and orgasm. A high-tone pelvic floor can also cause constipation with or without painful bowel movements.

5.2.1 Consequences of Stiff Pelvic Floor Muscles (High-Tone Dysfunction)

PFMs that are chronically tight or stiff pull and strain their relationships with other structures, including muscles, ligaments, bones, and fascia resulting in an imbalance (usually increase) of pressure on neighboring structures such as the bladder, prostate, and rectum, impacting proper function and blood flow. Lower urinary tract symptoms associated with HTD include voiding frequently, urgency, stress incontinence, pelvic pain, and dyspareunia.[74] Stiff, nonrelaxing PFMs can lead to pain with vaginal penetration (vaginismus), building arousal, or orgasm. Painful anismus and constipation with or without painful bowel movements are common with HTD. This high-tone state of the PFM's can also manifest in:

- Fear of relationships
- Fear of pain with intercourse
- Chronic pain behaviors
- Double urination

6 Common Forms of Incontinence

The most common forms of incontinence discussed in this book are stress, urge, and mixed incontinence. Bed-wetting (nocturnal enuresis), dribbling of urine, and the inability to empty the bladder (retention) are other forms of incontinence. It is essential to understand the difference between stress urinary incontinence (SUI) and urge urinary incontinence (UUI) because their treatments are very different. With UUI, the sudden, unstoppable loss of urine is sensed, whereas, with SUI, there is no immediate urge to urinate. The most common underlying cause of SUI is a weak sphincter muscle and pelvic floor.

Some of the exercises may improve these conditions. They may also be beneficial in cases of nocturia (having to get up at night to urinate).

6.1 Mixed Incontinence

The combination of stress and urge incontinence is called mixed incontinence (MI). Frequently the symptoms of one of the types of incontinence are more dominant than the other. Clients with MI can leak with coughing and sneezing as well as experience urgency and its related consequences.

6.2 Stress Urinary Incontinence

In many patients, stress urinary incontinence (SUI) is associated with urgencies, and therapists should, therefore, inquire about urgency symptoms. SUI is the most common form of incontinence in women under the age of 60 years, accounting for 50% of the known cases.[41] The underlying cause can be a weakness of the bladder sphincter muscles or weakness of the pelvic floor or both.

Weakness of the pelvic floor muscles as a result of pregnancy, childbirth, and aging is the top reason for stress incontinence (weakness and urgency with or without loss of urine). Common symptoms are loss of urine when coughing, sneezing, running, and jumping. In severe cases, loss of urine also occurs when turning in bed or without performing any specific activity.

The patient's history may be significant: the birth of a massive child, difficult prolonged labor, and episiotomy can all impact the support structures. SUI can result in men from not only prostate surgery, but also poor posture and incorrect body mechanics, for example, when lifting heavy objects or working in a garden. Faulty breathing techniques (pushing on to the pelvic floor during breathing) when lifting, combined with weak pelvic floor muscles can also lead to leakage of urine. SUI is often combined with UUI.

6.3 Urgency Urinary Incontinence

Urgency "urinary incontinence" (UUI) describes the urge to go to the bathroom instantly. Sometimes the urgency can be so great that it results in loss of urine before the individual reaches the toilet. It can be part of stress incontinence and also for other reasons.

Some clients do not experience urgencies during the day, but only at night. The reverse. of this can also be true. Consideration of working postures/habits, day time activities/behaviors, and the effect of the positional change of the pelvic structures due to gravity can provide pertinent information.

Having a patient keep a diary is the easiest way to obtain information about individual habits. For example, the patient writes down for 3 days, including one on the weekend, how much fluid (and what kind) is taken in, and how frequently and how much are expelled. Especially with clients who suffer from urgencies, counting the seconds of urination may be helpful to find out about a voiding pattern. Even though this is by no means an exact measure, because the strength of the stream also plays a role, it provides individuals with information about their behavior or habits. If, for example, a person can urinate for 15 seconds after waking, the same person may learn that the bladder is sending out an incorrect signal when the urgency to urinate during the day results in a 5-second urination. This error may be a sign of a "misbehaving" bladder. Patients can develop the understanding that regaining control of the situation is possible. Also, I treat my clients with connective tissue manipulation (CTM), which helps balance the autonomic nervous system and visceral mobilization of the kidneys. It appears to improve the decrease of urgencies and frequencies further. Exercises that may help are described in Part II of this book.

If the bladder does not empty well when in a hurry or when not sitting down properly on the toilet seat, this sometimes results in a "double urination," lasting for example 10 seconds.

When getting up a second urination is required for 5 more seconds. This situation could be a signal that the pelvic floor is not sufficiently relaxed when emptying the bladder. A "double urination" with two double-digit numbers could indicate high residuals and urine backing up into the kidneys, and a doctor should further evaluate this.

Children with bladder problems can color in a voiding diary, marking various events in different colors.

Case Examples

- A 25-year-old client was unable to sleep for 2 years because he had the urgency to urinate up to 14 times every night (no medication helped). He had normal voiding during the day. Finally, he was sent for treatment. I listened to his problems, and after explaining the function of the bladder and discussing drinking habits and nutrition, I instructed him to count every time during urination and write down how long he had to count during the daytime and also at night. With a full bladder (approximately 450 mL), the patient could count to 20 to 30. He understood then that there was no real need to urinate all night. After the first visit, he urinated 8 to 10 times, the next week he was down to 6 times, then to 4 times; on the 6th and 7th weeks he voided 3 times. In the first 8 weeks a stress situation made him urinate six times, and then he was down to one to two times. The client was sleeping again, could resume running and baseball training, and did not require any medicine.

- Another client, a retired professional, had the opposite problem. He had to urinate about every half an hour during the day, but not at night. Again, I let him count while urinating first time in the morning when his bladder was full. He soon understood that he did not have to urinate every 30 minutes in the daytime and quickly restored regular voiding during the daytime. Of course, it helps to find out what could have caused frequent urination. In the first client, a stressful event had started the problem. The second client was a very rational person who decided to stop going to the bathroom all the time when he understood how much his bladder could hold.

6.4 Urinary Frequency

The term "urinary frequency" (UF) is used when a client runs to the toilet up to 20 times. It is an acquired habit for various reasons, or the client may suffer from painful bladder syndrome where the lining of the inside can have ulcers, and filling the bladder causes pain. These clients may void up to 20 times per day. Weak pelvic floor muscles can lead to instability of the bladder (detrusor instability) and result in the frequent urge to have to go to the bathroom. Bladder infections can cause increased sensitivity and engender urge frequency. Poor regulation of all or some of the reflexes involved in emptying the bladder can also be a cause. Interstitial cystitis, also known as bladder pain syndrome, causes clients to urinate up to 20 times during the day because the lining within the bladder wall can have ulcers, scars, and stiffness, which cause pain when the bladder expands. Clients with urgencies can have difficulty with many foods that irritate the bladder (or the bowel). Best current information and recommendation for treatment and a special diet can be acquired from the Interstitial Cystitis Association. The goal of the physical therapist is to help to increase carefully the volume the bladder could hold.

6.5 Toilet Habits and Training

Individuals who have problems relaxing the pelvic floor muscles should sit properly on the toilet seat, not sit on the edge or in a half-squatting position. In these positions, the pelvic floor muscles are not able to relax properly. Children or people with short legs need a stool to rest their feet on.

6.5.1 Elimination Strategies for Difficult Bowel Emptying

In order to eliminate feces while sitting on the toilet, it may be helpful to move the upright trunk forward and backward while consciously relaxing the pelvic floor muscles. The pelvis can be tilted forward during inhalation and backward during exhalation to stimulate bowel movement. Sometimes turning the trunk to the right (or left) side may assist movement of the feces into the colon (see ▶ Fig. 9.6, ▶ Fig. 9.7, ▶ Fig. 9.8).

It is important to relax the pelvic floor muscles while using the pressure from the contraction of the abdominal muscles to help eliminate feces. Squeezing out stool may have an adverse effect and contribute to hemorrhoids. After eliminating the feces, it is advisable to activate the anus approximately 10 times by pulling it up and inward and then wipe. This strengthens the sphincter muscles and reduce the amount of toilet paper used when the sphincter anus has closed again.

Attention should be paid to signals from the body for bowel elimination, which are often suppressed. Rearranging daily routines may solve this problem. Normally the desire to defecate usually occurs 15 to 30 minutes after the first big meal. Clients with difficulty should get up earlier in the morning so they can eliminate feces before they leave the house. When the desire to eliminate daily is postponed (e.g., when driving on the freeway), the stool hardens, and elimination is more difficult, and it can lead to hemorrhoids.

6.5.2 Voiding Diary and Counting Seconds

Having a patient to keep a diary is the easiest way to obtain information about individual habits. For example, the patient tracks for 3 days how much and what type of fluid are taken in. They also track how frequently and how much are expelled (see Voiding Diary, Appendix E [p. 109]).

Especially with patients who suffer from urgencies, counting the seconds of urination may help the client discover a voiding pattern. Even though this is by no means an exact measure, because the strength of the stream also plays a role, it provides individuals with information about their behavior or habits. If a person can urinate for 15 seconds after waking, they can learn that the bladder is sending out a wrong signal when the urge to urinate during the day is followed by only a 5-second urination. This error may be a sign of a "misbehav-

ing" bladder, and understanding it may help regain control of the situation. Exercises that may help are described in Chapter 9 (p. 29).

If the bladder does not empty well when in a hurry or not sitting correctly on the toilet seat, this can result in a "double urination." In such cases, 10 seconds of urine flow is followed by 5 more seconds. This could be a signal that the pelvic floor is not sufficiently relaxed when emptying the bladder. A "double urination" with two double-digit numbers could indicate high residuals and urine backing up into the kidneys, and this should undoubtedly be further evaluated by a doctor.

Children with bladder problems can color in a voiding diary, marking various events in different colors.

Case Example

A child with an incomplete injury to her spinal cord following an accident was asked to mark the diary with different colors. She was taught to do this when she had the feeling of wanting to go to the bathroom when her residual urine in the bladder was low. The diary became an incentive to empty the bladder well and to create awareness of the bowel reflex.

Attention should be paid to signals from the body for bowel elimination, which are often suppressed. Rearranging daily routines may solve this problem.

If pelvic floor treatments are not adequate, physician intervention may be necessary and can work in conjunction with specialized pelvic floor physical therapy. Potential treatments include medication, Botox bladder injections, vaginal electrical stimulation, percutaneous tibial nerve stimulation, and sacral neuromodulation.

7 Medications, Nutrition, Intake of Fluid, and Adequate Hydration

What a client eats and drinks can have both direct and indirect effects on bowel and bladder symptoms. Continence can be impacted both positively and negatively by the diet. Medications can have an impact as well, so tracking responses to what one eats and drinks can provide much insight. There exists the potential for improvements of some of the continence-related challenges with proper understanding of the diet.

7.1 Medications and Continence

Over-the-counter medications for the treatment of colds or allergies can influence the pelvic floor muscles, as can some drugs for depression, high blood pressure, Parkinson's disease, and heart conditions. Some medications increase relaxation of the pelvic floor; others help to suppress urgencies; often though the side effects are very unpleasant, for example, dryness of the mouth, constipation, and dizziness. Diuretics can cause frequent urination and leakage if the pelvic floor muscles are weak.

Medication for treatment of incontinence and urgencies can be useful but may have side effects as described above. Some patients need to take medicines for treatment of depression, high blood pressure, and incontinence. It is essential to understand the mechanisms of the drug's actions to anticipate possible side effects on the pelvic floor muscles or bladder function. Discussion with a doctor can guide in proper planning and setting expectations.

With the help of the exercises in this book, continence is possible in many cases without having to resort to medication and managing urgencies. One may develop the ability to improve continence even if medications described above are required for a medical condition.

7.2 Nutritional Intake

Many foods can act as stimulants to the bladder, and individuals affected by incontinence should try to eliminate some of these irritants to find out if it makes a difference. Coffee and carbonated drinks are well-known diuretics, which is highlighted by the following story:

> ### Case Example
>
> A client came for treatment because of leakage from the bladder and urgencies 10 years after prostate surgery. He did very well after a few treatments, and his urgency to go to the bathroom frequently no longer appeared to be a problem. On one of his last visits, he told me: "I did well until yesterday when I went to a movie with a friend. I had to hurry to get to the bathroom." "What did you do with your friend before the movie?" I inquired. "Well, we sat down and had a Coke." The client then realized that the combination of caffeine and carbonation was undoubtedly not a tremendous pre-movie drink for a man suffering from urgencies.

Some clients react to artificial sweeteners, citrus fruits, and almost all respond to alcohol, which is also considered a diuretic. Spicy foods can cause problems. Therefore, it may be helpful to observe how the body reacts to certain foods and keep track of what was eaten the day before.

Common bladder irritants include:
- Alcohol
- Carbonated beverages
- Chocolate
- Citrus juice
- Coffee and tea
- Corn syrup
- Cranberries
- Fruit (e.g., apples, citrus)
- Honey
- Milk
- Spicy foods
- Sugar and artificial sweeteners
- Tomatoes
- Vinegar

Anyone with bowel dysfunction should make sure that his or her diet is well balanced and contains fiber. If necessary, a consultation with a nutritionist is an option.

Daily fluid intake should be six to eight glasses of water a day or approximately 2.5 L (just over half a gallon). Urination should be roughly every 2 to 4 hours, which is six to eight times a day. It is typical for some adults over 50 years to get up once at night to urinate.

Part 2

Treatment Options and Exercises

8 The Pelvic Floor—The Almost Forgotten Muscle Group

Many men and women exercise in health clubs or at home to keep in good physical shape. However, there is a group of muscles that are often left untrained even though they are vital to our well-being and our physical and sexual health. Weak or deconditioned pelvic floor muscles (PFMs) can cause back and pelvic pain, incontinence, and decreased libido during sexual intercourse. The muscles lie invisible in the center of the body and cover the opening of the bony structure of the pelvis between the sitting bones, tailbone, and pubic bone. They have the thickness of a hand, are shaped like a hammock, and are called the *PFMs.*

Strengthening these muscles, as one would exercise the biceps of the arm or the quadriceps of the leg, can improve physical and sexual health and may empower women and men to enhance their self-esteem and confidence. "When I discovered my pelvic floor muscles, I got the 'tiger feeling,'" the Swiss author Cantieni states in her book *Tiger Feeling*, which is about sensual training of the pelvic floor.[7,8,9,10]

German physical therapists Tanzberger and Heller developed pelvic floor exercises using a Swiss ball. This innovation has helped many individuals suffering from the consequences of weak PFMs.[31,68] The exercises described in this book are based on their work and the work of Klein-Vogelbach (1990a), a physical therapist from Switzerland who was my mentor and who also inspired Mrs. Tanzberger. When I returned to the USA in 1984 and joined the women's health section of the American Physical Therapy Association (APTA), I told my colleagues that there are exercises that are fun and motivating for the clients, and could also be practiced with a Swiss ball. I was asked to teach a pelvic floor Swiss ball exercise class at a preconference class at their next meeting. The course was well received by the many therapists who only knew Kegel exercises for the pelvic floor. For many years I then taught classes in different US states or hospitals and also taught classes based on motor learning.

8.1 Medical Examination

The first step to take when suffering from back pain, sexual dysfunction, or loss of urine or bowel control is to consult a doctor. There are many reasons why problems arise. The reason may be a weak pelvic floor, and in some cases, it could be an underlying medical or neurological condition. For example, an infection, which can irritate the bladder and cause urgencies and loss of urine, or perhaps bladder stones, or a lumbar structure pressing on a pelvic nerve, or problems due to diabetes, or even cancer. A thorough evaluation and additional treatment may be indicated, regardless of whether the problem originated from the back of the pelvic floor.

8.2 Safety Precautions

- The exercises should be done after confirmation by a physical therapist or after evaluation by the appropriate healthcare provider that they may be beneficial (and not detrimental) to one's condition.
- The exercises should be done in a safe environment to eliminate the risk of falling, especially if there is a history of osteoporosis.
- Individuals with poor balance or judgment need supervision while doing exercises with a Swiss ball.
- Damaged or punctured balls should never be repaired nor reused.
- Balls should be pumped up according to manufacturers' recommendations only.
- Exercises should be done on a low-pile carpet or a mat. To avoid slipping, it is advisable to wear shoes with a good grip.
- For activities performed sitting on the Swiss ball, the ball should be firm to limit contact of the body and ball with the area between the sitting bones, tailbone, and pubic bone.
- Not everyone needs to do all these exercises. Exercises can be adapted to personal needs or skills.

The following exercises and treatment suggestions are designed to help restore continence and fitness of the pelvic floor. These exercises may also be beneficial for individuals who suffer from fecal incontinence, urgencies, or hemorrhoids.

8.3 The Evolution of Traditional Pelvic Floor Exercises

New approaches to exercise design for this group integrates knowledge of neurophysiology and how one learns motor tasks, which can improve the fitness of the PFMs. The exercises are fun and can help to strengthen these essential muscles within our skeletal system as well as improve fitness of the entire center of the body, the pulmonary diaphragm, and the abdominal and back muscles.

Dr. Kegel's discovery that the PFMs contract like other muscles[36] led to his creation of "traditional" pelvic floor exercises. He recognized that the pelvic floor is trainable. Dr. Kegel first prescribed his exercises in 1948 and is considered a pioneer. Originally intended as a treatment for weak PFMs, women were instructed to squeeze the muscles around the anus and the vagina 300 times a day and continue with 80 daily squeezes for the rest of their lives. Frequently patients gave up exercising; the functional link was missing, and the muscles trained in isolation. Today, Kegel exercises are still the most commonly prescribed exercises despite the fact that most of the women treated using this approach had limited or no lasting success.[5]

8.4 The Emergence of Functional Pelvic Floor Exercises

The PFMs are a complicated group which do not work in isolation. They work in a synergistic pattern with muscles of the trunk and legs, and provide stability of the pelvic floor and the viscera (inner abdominal organs). After injury, illness, postural problems, or decreased mobility, changes in sensory awareness, emotional state, and even motor control may be lost. It is best to restore the functions before they lead to faulty movement patterns.

Motor relearning takes days, weeks, or months with repetitive practice to maintain the skill. The human nervous system can learn and modify motor programs. Neuroplasticity then molds the brain through interactions of tissues, neurons, and chemicals to make adaptations to the central nervous system (CNS). It takes weeks, months, or years to adapt, and depends on the ability and motivation of the individual to learn and integrate these adaptions. Procedural learning is "knowing how" I can get to the bathroom without losing urine. Declarative knowledge is "knowing that" I have to do deep breathing and fast fiber training (quick contractions of the PFMs) before I get out of the car to reach the bathroom safely.

Carefully listening to the client and designing an exercise program that helps and motivates the client can create meaning for the client. For example, if the client must lift heavy objects, this is practiced activating the slow fibers more frequently than the fast fibers. This sequence makes sense because it takes longer to bend over and lift a heavy object. If coughing or sneezing happens a lot, fast fibers are the most relevant and have to be trained. If a client has difficulty to initiate urination, he/she has to practice breathing and relaxation of his/her PFMs.

Exercises have to be individualized and done daily. Clients are encouraged to practice the training activities throughout the day in the situations where they have challenges. This experience can be empowering when coupled with their "why" behind correcting these problems in the first place. Motivation is of utmost importance to achieve a meaningful goal. For example, if a client desires to work in the garden or hit a tennis ball without urine leakage, connecting these activities to the necessary exercises reinforces their importance. Disrupted sleep due to urinary frequency can be a strong motivator to exercise consistently and maintain compliance as the impact is readily experienced. The ability to relax the pelvic floor enough to empty the bladder without straining has biomechanical as well as psychological control implications. Control of urgencies and frequent urination in order to sleep through the night creates a meaningful "cause and effect" relationship with daily exercises. A faulty movement pattern has to be "unlearned." The patient can learn to gently feel a contraction of the PFMs in different directions (tail bone toward pubic bone—back to front) or pull the sitting bones from the sides toward the middle. The client then can learn to correct the breathing dysfunction and then refine the exercises (see ▶ Fig. 9.2, ▶ Fig. 9.3, and ▶ Fig. 9.4). Do them together, as shown in this section, to guide the clients toward their goal.

Also, there are three main home-based approaches to pelvic floor exercises aimed at improving the health and flexibility of the PFMs which can be useful:
- Active stretching via breathing-visualization and relaxation with external perineal input (i.e., ball sit).
- Trigger point release via internal massage.
- Focused mental relaxation exercises, with or without gentle vibration, can help those who experience involuntary muscle spasm.

8.5 Individual Objectives

- To *achieve* sensory awareness of the PFMs.
- To *restore* coordination of the PFMs with the pulmonary diaphragm.
- To *coordinate* the activity of the muscles surrounding the pelvic floor with the function of the PFMs.
- To *train* the muscle fibers in different planes of movement.
- To *strengthen* fast and slow muscle fibers of the pelvic floor.
- To *train* functional activities.

> **Note**
>
> Think of "ARMS": Awareness, Relaxation, Motor Control, and Strengthening.

9 Sensory Awareness—Feeling the Pelvic Floor

The sensory system "drives" the motor system: Touching or tapping a muscle increases afferent sensory information, which informs the cerebellum that the muscle may have to do a task. Before beginning these exercises, it is vital to understand where the invisible pelvic floor muscles (PFMs) are and to feel them. The anal sphincter is at the end of the digestive tract, which begins at the mouth. The muscle can be contracted in the same way as one would pucker the mouth (▶ Fig. 9.1).

Awareness increases by touching a muscle, such as the anal sphincter, and feeling its contraction, which may also contribute to increased intensity of the contraction. Very faint at first and barely palpable, the client eventually elicits the contraction by visualization only.

The brain is very powerful and will adjust the contraction depending on what the client visualizes. For example, a client elicits a measurably different contraction according to whether he or she imagines holding a lentil or a marble with the sphincter muscle. The ability to contract a muscle in many different ways improves skill and awareness, as does practice. Performing variations of the same exercise and repeated practice are the fundamental tenets of motor learning. Once imprinted on the brain, these skillful movements can be retrieved quickly, whenever needed. The quality of contraction of a muscle is at least as important as its quantity.

The muscles of the mouth, for example, can be puckered by sucking up fluid through a straw, blowing out candles, spitting out cherry pits, blowing soap bubbles, or bubbles from gum, kissing, or saying words beginning with "p." The same concept applies to the PFMs. The knowledge of exercising PFMs in different combinations (i.e., with breathing, use of the abdominal or back muscles, or coughing or sneezing) is integrated through palpation and sensory awareness. This activity helps the clients develop "automatic" responses in place of reactive ones. The clients know they have achieved the necessary skill when the PFMs automatically contract while lifting, going upstairs, coughing, etc. If the sensory awareness of the PFMs is intact and the strength restored, individuals may able to activate the pelvic floor when it is necessary automatically.

> **Note**
>
> The first step is to learn how to feel the muscle contractions!

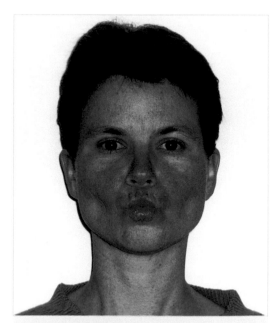

Fig. 9.1 The anal sphincter can be puckered similarly to how one puckers the mouth.

9.1 Awareness through Touching (Palpation)

Touching is a powerful tool for reeducating muscles. Once we have perceived a muscle contraction and make the connection with the brain, we increase our ability to contract a muscle correctly and to distinguish between a weak and strong contraction.

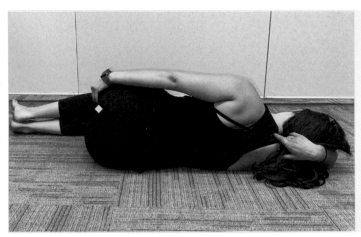

Fig. 9.2 The contraction should be felt at the fingertips only.

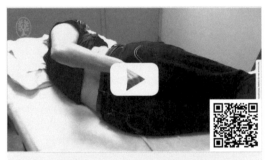

Video 9.1 Fascia self-mobilization at tail bone in sidelying position

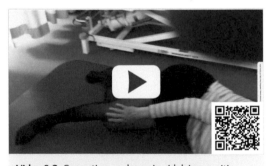

Video 9.2 Correcting prolapse in sidelying position

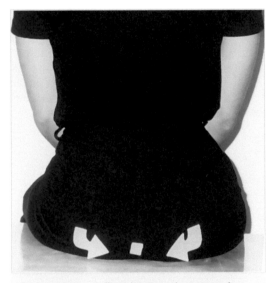

Fig. 9.3 Imagine pulling the sitting bones together.

9.1.1 Exercises in Side-Lying Position

- Place one hand over the buttock with the fingertips at the anus or perineal area (i.e., between the anus and the urethra).
- The tightening of the center muscles should be felt at the fingertips only (▶ Fig. 9.2) (▶ Video 9.1 and ▶ Video 9.2).

9.1.2 Exercises Standing or Seated with Feet Resting on the Floor

- Touch the sitting bones on the right and left sides with both hands and then imagine pulling them together.
- Feel the tightening of the muscles in the center of the seat around the anal sphincter (▶ Fig. 9.3).
- With one hand, touch the tail bone from behind, and with the other hand, the pubic bone from the front.
- A slight contraction can be felt at the side of the tip of the tail bone when you imagine pulling the tail bone toward the navel (▶ Fig. 9.4).

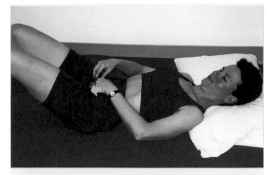

Fig. 9.5 Palpate contraction of the pelvic floor muscles and transversus abdominis muscle at the inside of the pubic bone.

9.2 Awareness through Visualization

Imagination is a powerful tool and very helpful, especially when training invisible muscles such as those which make up the pelvic floor.[64]

9.2.1 Exercises

- Visualize pulling the sitting bones together. You can also imagine pulling the tail bone forward toward the pubic bone (see anatomy drawings in Chapter 2 [p. 6]).
- Visualize picking up a tissue, lentil, raisin, blueberry, and marble with the anus, vagina, or urethra and feel the contraction of the PFMs.
- Visualize the PFMs opening and closing like a flower.
- Pretend to squeeze out a sponge.

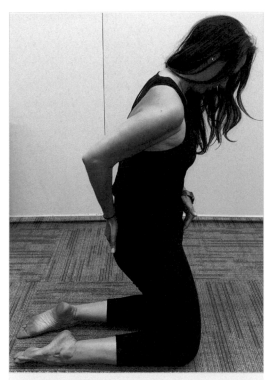

Fig. 9.4 Touch the tail bone and pubic bone. Imagine pulling the tail bone forward.

9.1.3 Exercises Lying on the Back

> **Note**
>
> Only people with a strong PFM may be able to perform these exercises.

- With the fingertips, feel a contraction of the transversus abdominus below the belly on the inside of the pelvic rim (iliac crest); imagine the right and left rims moving toward each other.

The close relationship between the PFMs and the abdominal muscles is best palpated in this area. Connection to the transverse abdominus and the oblique abdominal muscles is more accessible to palpation when exhaling (place fingers just below the rib cage). The cue of flattening the abdomen without increased flattening of the lumbar spine and contracting the PFMs (▶ Fig. 9.5).

> **Note**
>
> Visualizing and sensing contraction of the anal sphincter is felt at the anus, while contraction of the vagina and urethra can be felt more in the front of the seat.

Sex shops have long recognized the importance of sensory awareness, selling all kinds of gadgets that enhance the feeling of the pelvic floor. Normal sensation with awareness and positive feedback drives the motor system, that is, it improves the performance of the muscles.

Excellent performance of the PFMs provides continence and can enhance sexual pleasure.

9.3 Awareness through Feeling by Touching

The following section describes exercises that can improve the sensory awareness of the PFMs through feeling with or without touching.

Coughing increases intra-abdominal pressure and can cause leakage of urine when the load or pressure bears down into the pelvic floor. The downward movement of the pelvic floor is felt. This downward movement is limited when the PFMs contract before coughing or sneezing.

9.3.1 Exercises

- Cough while sitting upright and feel the downward movement of the pelvic floor in the center of the seat.
- Cough while leaning forward or backward and explore how the response movement is more intense in the front or the back of the pelvic floor.
- Cough touching the perineal area while lying on the back or side, with and without tightening of the PFMs.

- Palpate and pucker the anal sphincter in side-lying position, then tighten the buttock muscles (gluteus maximus), then keep the anus puckered while relaxing the buttock muscles.

Feel the difference: When contracting the PFMs alone (see ▶ Fig. 9.2), the buttock muscles remain soft; the contraction can only be felt at the fingertips. If the buttock muscles are in contraction, the muscle tightness can also be felt with the hand.

Pearl

Clients who have experienced sexual abuse may not "feel" where an assailant touched them. The client has to relearn what feels pleasurable by touching themselves in body parts they have ignored. The therapist can help the client to restore feeling their body—with their consent—to feel different materials gently placed on areas of his/her body. With closed eyes, the client can learn to identify the objects (silk scarf, postcard, etc.). The clients also may have to learn the functions of bowel and bladder again.

9.4 Additional Possibilities for Feeling the Pelvic Floor Muscle

9.4.1 Lying on the Back

- Bend your knees, keep your feet on the floor, and spread your knees apart.
- Touch the perineal area (between anus and vagina) with the right and left hands, just in front of the anus, while breathing in and out.
- Feel the downward movement of the pelvic floor during inhalation. Trying to feel the movement or action without touching the area enhances sensory awareness.

Note

In women with scars in the pelvic area, such as from birth injury (e.g., episiotomy or accidents), one side may not move as well as the other as a result of the trauma. Gentle massage and conscious breathing into the area can improve the mobility of the pelvic floor.

9.4.2 Lying on the Stomach

- Touch your buttock muscles and feel the tightening of the PFMs by puckering anus, vagina, and urethra.
- Tense the buttock (gluteal) muscles (which are felt under the hands) and then try to relax the buttock muscles before relaxing the PFMs in the center of the seat.
- Repeat the PFM contraction without tensing the buttock to increase awareness of the PFM.

> **Pearl**
>
> Splash water with the hand or using a showerhead onto the pelvic floor. Alternatively, a wet towel can be pressed onto the center of the seat or can be used to dab it. This method activates the afferent input to the brain from temperature receptors in the skin.

9.5 Awareness Training with a Partner

- Sensory awareness improves with appropriate tactile stimulation. For example, a partner could trace letters or numbers with the fingertip on the perineal area, and guesses can be made with closed eyes what has been written.
- The perineal area can be gently stroked with a silk scarf or gently brushed to enhance the awareness of light touch.
- Women can place a finger between the labia on the opening of the urethra or vagina and feel a faint contraction when "puckering." Place one or two fingers in the vagina, pretend to "pick up a raisin" or tighten the vagina around the fingers, and feel the contraction of the PFMs.
- During intercourse, women can try to tighten the muscles of the vagina around the penis.
- Men should be able to palpate the contraction of their PFMs between the anus and the urethra. Pucker the anal sphincter muscle in the back, or pretend to squirt the last drop of urine out of the urethra, which can be felt more in the front of the seat.
- During PFM training, the contraction of the PFMs always precedes any activity of the surrounding muscles.

9.6 Awareness through Hearing (Auditory Input)

This form of sensory awareness is especially crucial for individuals who suffer from urgencies and frequent urination. The many reflexes from the bladder to the brain and spinal cord may be functioning improperly. The result is a feeling of having to urinate, although, in actuality, this may not be true. Auditory awareness can help individuals to get to know their bladder habits; this awareness can then be applied to correct problems.

> **Case Example**
>
> A male client developed the habit of going to the bathroom more than 30 times in 24 hours. (It is reasonable to go about 6 to 8 times during the day, and with older individuals up to 2 times at night.) His habit of frequent urination began after he passed a kidney stone. The doctor had told him to go to the bathroom often, and he had taken the advice literally. Of course, the doctor did not expect the man to go to the toilet every half hour or more, day and night.
>
> The patient practiced counting and listening to how many seconds he was urinating. The goal was to learn that 6 seconds of urination could not possibly mean that the bladder was full. The bladder had adopted a habit of frequent urination and may have shrunk as well. Over several weeks of training, the man's condition improved; urination took place every 2 to 3 hours during the day and twice during the night without any adverse effect on the kidneys. He was encouraged to delay the urination gradually to allow the bladder to increase the volume it could hold.

Even though the amount of urine flow per second may vary considerably, everyone can become aware of the pattern. Most adults may urinate for 12 to 15 seconds when the bladder is full, sometimes more in the morning after sleeping through the night. This pattern is variable depending on the amount of fluid consumed within a specific timeframe. Whether urine is "pressed out" or "flows out" of the bladder in a relaxed state without increasing intra-abdominal pressure also affects urination time.

> **Pearl**
>
> Men should urinate in a continuous stream. If men have to think about emptying their bladder or experience dribbling urine, an evaluation by a doctor is likely necessary.

Men, women, and teenagers if they have a bladder problem should:

- Listen to the urine flow and count how long urination lasts to create awareness of the pattern of the bladder. Does the urine flow easily? Is it necessary to press it out? Is it an interrupted stream? How many seconds does urination last after a night's sleep and how long it is during the day?
- Individuals experiencing double urination can double count each time they urinate while relaxing the PFMs by breathing calmly during urination. For example, 10/5 double count is when, after emptying the bladder for 10 seconds, there is a second trickle of 5 seconds. Another suggestion is to lean and tilt the pelvis slightly forward to position the urethra better for urination (more natural if the feet on the floor are not close together).
- Learn not to rush in the bathroom. The goal is not to have to sit down a second time.
- See a doctor for an evaluation if there is any doubt about the condition.
- Do not move or walk during a moment of urgency, or it may become uncontrollable. Stop moving and try some quick contractions of the PFMs and abdominal breathing exercises to relax.

> **Pearl**
>
> Teenagers who suffer from giggle incontinence can train and use the fast-fiber muscles with quick contractions when they are about to laugh and then relax when finished giggling.

9.7 Awareness Training for Fecal Urgencies and Constipation

A person with fecal urgencies and constipation needs to learn to be aware of the reflexes that create an urgency to empty the bowel. The urgency to empty the bowel occurs approximately 10 to 30 minutes, sometimes up to an hour, after the first big meal. This urgency may occur once or twice daily or every other day, depending on the speed of digestion. Versprille-Fischer reports that the urgency to defecate occurs each time a portion of the stool reaches the rectum. This urgency results in the relaxation of the PFMs.

Suppression of this reflex can occur from rushing around and not taking the time to use the toilet. In such cases, a person can adjust his or her lifestyle to accommodate a trip to the bathroom when the reflex occurs and restore this function. Retraining proper bowel evacuation is a process that may take many months, but the result is gratifying and rewarding.

> **Note**
>
> Versprille-Fischer states that it usually takes about 45 hours for food to pass through the digestive system.[71]

9.7.1 Exercises

- Learn to "feel" the reflex that occurs when the rectum fills and note when and how often it happens. A voiding diary can be used for this purpose (see Appendix [p. 109] and Chapter 6 [p. 22]).
- Arrange to be in a place where you can go to the bathroom when the urgency to evacuate the bowel occurs. This requires getting up earlier or arriving at work in time to go to the bathroom.
- Take time to relax the PFMs by sitting well supported on the toilet seat. Sitting on the edge of the seat does not help to relax the PFMs.
- Try some abdominal breathing exercises—tilting the pelvis forward during inhalation and backward during exhalation while flattening the lumbar spine. Repeat 5 to 10 times.

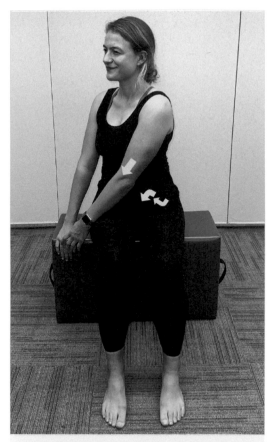

Fig. 9.6 Turning the trunk to the right or left side may facilitate movement of the bowel contents (*yellow arrows* indicate bowel journey) into the rectum (through increased abdominal pressure in an oblique direction).

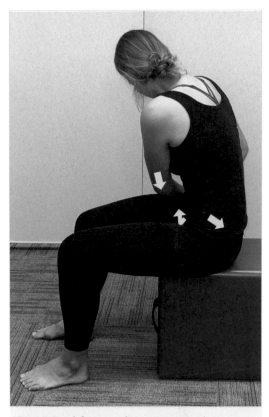

Fig. 9.7 For defecation, the rectum is in a better position when the pelvis is tilted backward.

- Do 5 to 10 quick, intense pucker movements of the anal sphincter before consciously relaxing the muscle.
- Tighten the anal sphincter muscle deliberately for 10 to 15 seconds and then relax it. This approach may help with a tight anal sphincter by fatiguing and thereby relaxing the muscle.
- During exhalation, the upright trunk can also turn to the left or right side. This increase of abdominal pressure in an oblique direction may assist the movement of the bowel contents into the colon (▶ Fig. 9.6 and ▶ Fig. 9.7).
- Try to relax the pelvic floor consciously. Do not try to squeeze the bowel out if the anal sphincter contracts as this could cause hemorrhoids.

Note

- For defecation, the colon is in a better position when the pelvis is tilted backward (▶ Fig. 9.7).
- For urination, the pelvis should be tilted slightly forward (▶ Fig. 9.8). Inhalation during the forward tilt may help relax the pelvic floor. Breathe normally without straining.
- If the fecal urge sensation occurs too frequently, breathing exercises, quick puckering, and self-relaxation may assist in readjusting it.
- Do not squeeze out bowel contents. It is better to activate bowel evacuation through movement.

All the exercises in this book are beneficial for various bladder problems. They can also improve bowel (fecal) continence and control of gas (flatus) as well as help individuals suffering from hemorrhoids.

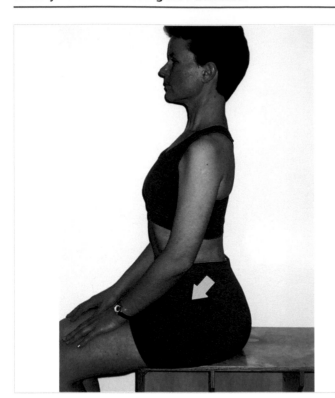

Fig. 9.8 For urination, the urethra is in a better position when the pelvis is tilted forward.

10 Exercises to Increase Sensory Awareness, Skill, and Coordination of Muscles Attached to the Pelvic Floor

The following exercises are based on the concepts of Cantieni,[10] Heller,[31] Tanzberger,[68] and Klein-Vogelbach. They can be done at any time anywhere, for example, while sitting in a car in a traffic jam, doing the dishes, watching TV, or taking an afternoon nap. They can be done seated with both feet on the ground, standing, sitting on your heels, or lying on one's side or back.

10.1 Exercises through Visualization Alone

- Visualize pulling your sitting bones (ischial tuberosities) together (see ▶ Fig. 9.3).
- Visualize pulling your tail bone (coccyx) toward your pubic bone (see ▶ Fig. 9.4).

- Visualize pulling your tail bone toward your left or right sitting bone.

10.2 Exercises Combining Visualization and Movement

- Pucker the anus, then lift up one sitting bone. Women can pretend to hold a raisin with the vagina, then lift up one sitting bone in sitting or standing position and lower it (▶ Fig. 10.1).
- Pucker the anal sphincter muscle at the back and pretend to tighten the urethra at the front. Move the sitting bone about 1 cm forward then backward (▶ Fig. 10.2). This activity can be done sitting, standing, or lying on the back with both legs bent.

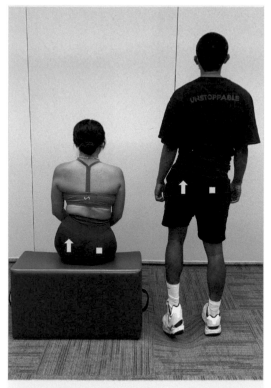

Fig. 10.1 Pucker your anal sphincter muscle and lift one sitting bone upward.

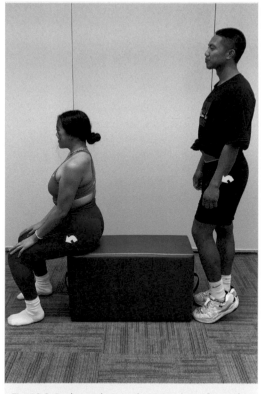

Fig. 10.2 Pucker and move the sitting bone forward.

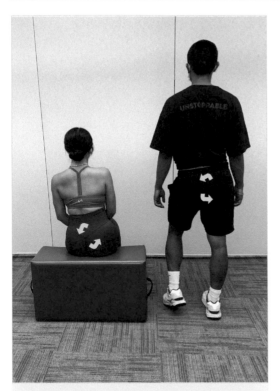

Fig. 10.3 Pucker and make a circle with one and then the other sitting bone.

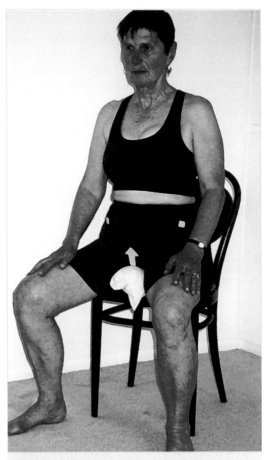

Fig. 10.4 Sit on a firm roll and visualize lifting the center of the seat from the roll.

- Pucker and visualize tightening the pelvic floor muscles. Make a circular movement with the sitting bones, forming the first half of the circle with one side and completing it with the other (► Fig. 10.3 and ► Video 11.3).
- Pucker the pelvic floor muscles and make a figure of "8," half with the right side and half with the left side.
- Pucker the pelvic floor muscles and make a figure of "8," first in a forward, then a backward direction, first with one then the other sitting bone.
- Find the tail bone with one hand and the pubic bone with the other; visualize pulling the tail bone toward the pubic bone during exhalation. Feel the pelvic floor muscles contract, then relax when exhaling and letting go of the contraction (see ► Fig. 9.4).
- Pretend or try to pick up a golf ball between the anus and urethra (perineal area). Alternatively,

sit on a firm roll and pretend to lift up the seat from the center of the roll (► Fig. 10.4).
- Sit on the floor with outstretched legs and "walk" forward or backward by moving the buttocks. At the same time, pucker the pelvic floor muscles and visualize tightening the sphincter around the urethra.

Note

In all the above exercises, women can visualize picking up a raisin with the vagina.

10.3 Exercises in Side-Lying Position

When exercising in the side-lying position, make sure that the movements come from the pelvis only. The chest and the knees should not move.

10.4 Exercises Lying on the Back with the Knees Bent and Apart

Exercise combining visualization and movement:

- Try moving the sitting bones up and down, forward and backward, in circles, and a figure of "8" while puckering and pretending to hold a raisin.

10.5 Sitting on the Heels, Kneeling, or Standing on the Hands and Knees

Exercises combining visualization and movement

> **Note**
>
> - All exercises can be coordinated by breathing out during puckering and breathing in during relaxation of the pelvic floor muscles.
> - As an additional benefit, these exercises are beneficial for gentle mobilization of the hip joints and the lumbar spine in all directions. The exercises primarily train the skill and coordination of all the muscles of the hip joint that attach to the pelvis. Likewise, the muscles of the lower abdomen and the trunk are trained in skill and coordination.

10.6 Exercises Seated on a Stool

10.6.1 Ball Sit Pelvic Floor Differentiation

Approaching the exercise with a sense of purpose improves contraction of the pelvic floor, increases awareness of anterior versus posterior floor bias, and is important for proper neuromuscular control and stability.

- Sit tall on a chair or perform one sustained 5-second pelvic floor contraction, and observe how it feels.
- Now, place a small ball (15–20 cm diameter) in the center of the triangle created by your pubic bone and sit bones (i.e., ischial tuberosities), making sure you feel equal weight throughout.
- Reach your arms forward, palms in.
- Sit on the ball for 30 seconds, working up to 60 seconds.
- Remove the ball, noticing how you feel (e.g., Do you feel like you're sitting in a hole?).
- Practice one slow contraction of your pelvic floor, first contracting the front, the back, and then the full floor. Assess how you feel—any differences?
- Do five fast pulse-like contractions coupled with quick exhales. Self-assess to see if you feel any different.
- Breathe naturally throughout, with an exhale on the quick pulses.
- This exercise can be modified by using a softer or larger ball, and/or lowering your hands to a Pilates long box to offset some of your weight.

> **Pearl**
>
> - If your clients experience a significant difference in their connection with the pelvic floor with this exercise, begin with it.

10.6.2 Seated Slow-Twitch Prep

- Sit tall on a chair, bench, or Pilates long box with your legs sit-bone distance apart and a ball between your knees.
- Reach your arms toward the front of the seat, activating your back muscles.
- Ground into your sit bones while reaching through the crown of your head with your pelvis in neutral.

- Press your feet into the floor and activate your hamstrings by energetically drawing your heels toward the chair or the Pilates long box.
- Draw the area of your pelvis between your sit bones towards each other and the pubic symphysis, then visualize connecting to the front (anterior) part of your pelvic floor (this will feel like 25%), and then engage your whole floor.
- Hold this sustained connection from your heels to the top of your head while contracting your pelvic floor for 5 seconds, then release for a full 10 seconds.
- Do five repetitions, breathing naturally throughout.

10.6.3 Seated Fast-Twitch Prep (The Setup Is the Same as Seated Slow-Twitch Prep)

- Exhale, drawing the bottom of your pelvis between your sit bones and pubic symphysis up, and engage your whole floor in a quick upward pulse with an immediate release.
- Do five repetitions, working up to 10 quick, coordinated pulses.

Note

- Teach the pelvic floor slow- and fast-twitch additions to any applicable exercise slowly.
- Make sure your client can always feel a relaxation phase of the pelvic floor between repetitions.
- The torso should not move up and down—this indicates overactivation of the gluteal muscles.
- This exercise can be modified by decreasing the pulses.

10.7 Frequency of Exercises

Throughout the day, try to create an awareness of your pelvic floor muscles by integrating 5 to 10 minutes of exercise into daily activities. As described previously, the muscles can contract while doing housework, sitting and watching TV, getting up from a seat, climbing stairs, or when stuck in traffic. Music with an even beat, for example, classical, jazz, or rap, makes these exercises fun.

Note

- Be cautious with frequency and intensity.
- Individuals with reduced awareness of their pelvic floor muscles can over-exercise. The focus of therapy should then be on relaxation or even fatiguing the pelvic muscles to enable the muscles to relax.
- Biofeedback may be required for the patient to learn to relax the pelvic floor or surrounding muscles.

10.8 Problems Caused by Hypertonic Muscles in the Pelvic Region

A client with pain during sexual intercourse (dyspareunia). The client was not aware of how difficult it was for her to relax the pelvic floor muscles. Even during biofeedback therapy, relaxation of the pelvic floor was a challenge. One day the client came to treatment after a treadmill test for her heart and told the therapist, "I'm exhausted from walking on the treadmill." For the first time, biofeedback measurements showed a total relaxation of the pelvic floor muscles. The client was advised to take a walk to fatigue her muscles before sexual intercourse. This activity led to an improvement in her condition.

A 53-year-old woman suffering from bladder prolapse and urinary incontinence with a history of cesarean delivery and hysterectomy. This client felt as if the bladder would fall out and was unable to relax the pelvic floor muscles. Intercourse was very painful, the muscles around the vagina were sore to touch, and she was unable to relax them (vaginismus). There was no history of sexual abuse.

During the evaluation, when on her back, the woman pressed her knees together. The muscles on the inside of her thighs (adductors) were very tight. The biofeedback probe, inserted while the patient was lying on her back, indicated that the pelvic floor muscles could not relax.

The client learned that she did not have to hold the bladder in by pressing her knees together. She was taught placing pillows under her buttocks. In this slanted position, with the head in a lower position, the client learned to relax her pelvic floor. Biofeedback confirmed the relaxation of the pelvic floor muscles in the slanted position. This alternative was a recommended option for intercourse.

Tight inner thigh muscles can cause pain in the center of the seat because they attach to the pubic bone. Therefore, equal attention was given to teaching the client how to relax her adductor muscles.[69] This type of relaxation is achieved by activating the external rotator and abductor muscles. The legs were pushed apart against the force of a tight elastic band.

11 Breathing Evaluation and Treatment of Breathing Dysfunction

Poor breathing patterns are so common that correct breathing (together with proper lifting) should be taught in kindergarten. Being told to "pull your stomach in" is probably a cause of faulty breathing patterns and "chest breathing." A shift in fashions and ideals is another contributing factor. Many men tend to pull in their stomach because it makes their chest appear larger. What is not commonly known is that it also makes the person more vulnerable to back problems because the lumbar spine loses its flexibility and the center of gravity changes with a raised chest.

The neck muscles can become tight because they cannot relax when used for breathing. Breathing primarily with the chest also prevents the pelvic floor muscles from working in union (synergy) with the pulmonary diaphragm.

11.1 Correction of Breathing Patterns

It is essential to correct faulty breathing patterns, not only for the sake of the pelvic floor muscles but also to decrease strain on the neck muscles. Good breathing may improve the oxy- gen supply to the pelvic floor through its many arteries. Oxygen is required for well-functioning muscles. Abdominal breathing coordinates the pulmonary diaphragm with the pelvic diaphragm and probably also helps to promote healthy bowel movements in the intestine. The abdominal and back muscles are trained when breathing is properly coordinated during activities such as walking, running, and lifting. Back injuries are prevented by a well-trained back and abdominal muscles, a well-aligned body, and muscles flexible enough to maintain good posture.

Breathing can be practiced sitting, standing, kneeling, or lying on the side or back.

11.2 Observation of the Shape of the Ribcage

Evaluating posture and the shape of the chest, ribcage, and abdomen may indicate possible respiratory problems.

- If the angle formed by the rib cage is greater than 90° this may indicate a breathing dysfunction, possibly secondary to weak oblique abdominal muscles and reduced downward movement of the pulmonary diaphragm.
- Horizontally positioned collar bones can indicate a possible postural and breathing problem. The scalene muscles may be tight. A therapist can further evaluate which corrective exercises may be necessary.
- Does the abdomen rise during inhalation and fall during exhalation?
- Does the movement come primarily from the chest or from the abdomen?
- In normal breathing the abdomen rises then the rib cage expands, the sternum lifts only slightly (▶ Fig. 11.1 and ▶ Fig. 11.2).

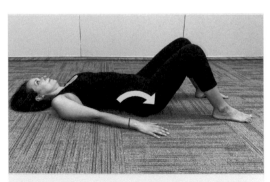

Fig. 11.1 During inhalation, the abdomen rises, and the chest expands only minimally.

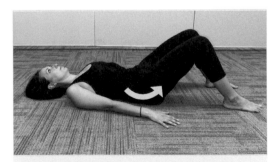

Fig. 11.2 The abdomen falls during exhalation.

- Breathing primarily with the chest is a common faulty breathing pattern.
- Another incorrect breathing pattern is to reverse the breathing, sucking the stomach in during inhalation and pushing it out during exhalation.
- Equally incorrect is correct rising of the abdomen during inhalation and flatting of the abdomen during exhalation but with "pouching" of the lower abdomen at the end of exhalation, usually with increase of abdominal pressure.

11.3 Exercises to Increase Sensory Awareness of the Breath and Its Connection to Pelvic Floor Function

- Place both hands flat on the abdomen, one above and one below the navel. Feel how the distance between the hands increases during inhalation and decreases during exhalation.
- Make a dome with the hands in front of the rib cage and visualize the diaphragm behind the rib cage. Flatten the hands downward during inhalation; return to the dome shape with exhalation (▶ Fig. 11.3 and ▶ Fig. 11.4).
- Let the fingertips of each hand rest under the rib cage. During inhalation, the fingers are moved forward and up by the diaphragm, if it expands correctly.
- "Grab" a skin fold of the abdomen and let it slip out of your hand by expanding the belly during inhalation.
- Place the fingertips below the rib cage and try panting, first fast, then slower, to "feel" the movement of the diaphragm.
- Place the fingers below the rib cage and breathe out against resistance of the glottis. Make a guttural sound in the back of the throat, such as the sound of static on the radio or telephone. Feel the oblique abdominal muscles contracting below the rib cage.
- Place the fingers below the tip of the sternum and feel the rectus abdominus muscle contracting when lifting the head and during exhalation. (This can also be felt above the pubic bone.)
- Place the fingers on the belly button. During exhalation, pretend to pull the belly button away from the fingers toward the spine. Feel the

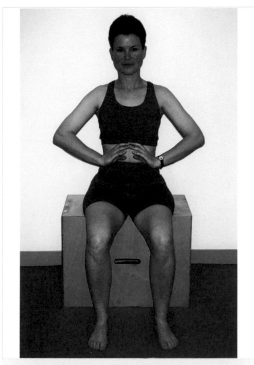

Fig. 11.3 The pulmonary diaphragm sits like a dome behind the rib cage.

contraction of the transversus abdominis, which helps to pull the pelvic diaphragm upward during its contraction.
- Place both hands on the abdomen and say explosive words such as "kick" or "cool" or pretend to spit out cherry pits. Feel the increase in abdominal pressure.
- Saying the words "kick" and "cool" forcefully has a similar effect to coughing or sneezing and can be used to retrain contraction of the pelvic floor before a cough or a sneeze.
- Understanding how to activate the different abdominal muscles helps the coordination of the pelvic floor muscles with the abdominal muscles.
- With flexion of the trunk, the angle of the rib cage widens, especially with activation of the rectus abdominis muscle. It also widens if the thorax is used primarily during respiration. Often it is then "stuck" in an inspiration position, and the client has to learn that the rib cage can also move downward.
- The external oblique abdominal muscles narrow the rib cage during exhalation.

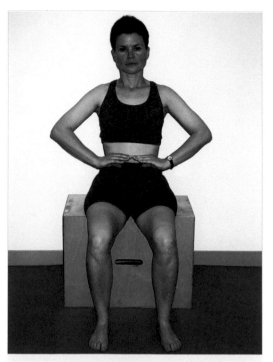

Fig. 11.4 During inhalation, the pulmonary diaphragm flattens and the abdomen protrudes.

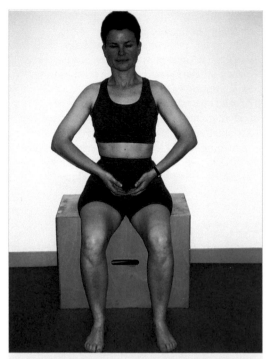

Fig. 11.5 The pelvic floor muscles move in a downward direction during inhalation.

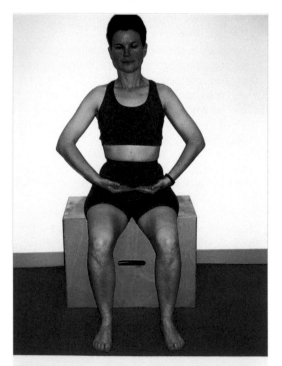

Fig. 11.6 During exhalation, the pelvic floor muscles contract in an upward direction.

Pearl

- The lower abdomen "shortens" during exhalation. If this initiates without increased flattening of the spine, the transverse abdominal muscle is activated.
- It is essential to know how to distinguish correct from incorrect breathing before coordinating breathing with pelvic floor contractions.
- Provided it does not cause any pain, the back can be arched slightly during inhalation and flattened during exhalation. This mobilizes the spine.
- Breathing can be practiced in various positions: lying on the back, side, or stomach; on hands and knees; sitting; or standing.
- Although breathing exercises and pelvic floor muscle contractions can be done separately, it is beneficial to practice them in coordination.
- During inhalation, the pelvic floor muscles relax with a minimal downward movement. During exhalation, they contract and move in an upward direction, assisted by contraction of the transversus abdominis muscle and possibly of the internal oblique muscles (▶ Fig. 11.5 and ▶ Fig. 11.6; ▶ Video 11.2 and ▶ Video 11.3).

(See ▶ Video 11.1, ▶ Video 11.4, ▶ Video 11.5, ▶ Video 11.6, ▶ Video 11.7, ▶ Video 11.8, and ▶ Video 11.9)

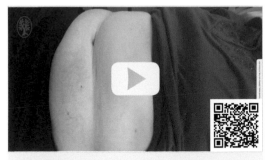

Video 11.1 Faulty breathing—"Grand Canyon"

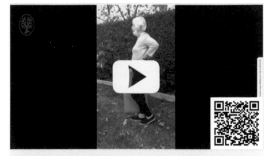

Video 11.2 Corrective standing coordination and balance of pelvic floor muscles

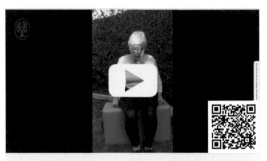

Video 11.3 Corrective sitting coordination and balance of pelvic floor muscles

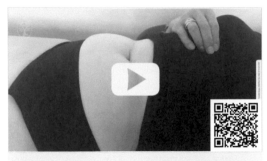

Video 11.4 Corrected "Grand Canyon" breathing after three treatments (note naval crease is improved)

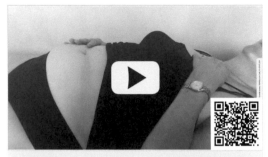

Video 11.5 Corrected "Grand Canyon" pattern after four treatments (note naval crease is diminished)

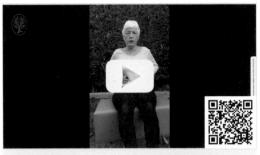

Video 11.6 Example of seated panting exercise correction

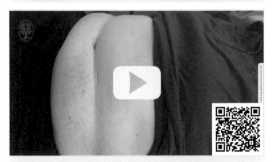

Video 11.7 Corrected "Grand Canyon" pattern in supine position

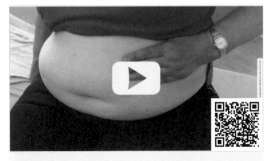

Video 11.8 Corrected "Grand Canyon" pattern in sitting position

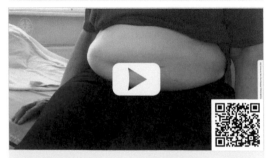

Video 11.9 Corrective breathing progression in sitting position

12 Treatment with Functional Exercises

There exist many applications of Pilates based exercises and breathwork, which are applicable to each of these treatment options. It is imperative to seek out and work with a trained practitioner who specializes not only in Pilates but its application to pelvic health.

The following exercises are based on the concepts of Heller,[31] Klein-Vogelbach,[39,40] and Tanzberger.[68]

12.1 Safety with Prop Usage

Before exercising with a ball, the safety precautions set out below should be observed:

- Provide a safe environment. Individuals who do not feel safe on a ball or who suffer from balance problems could use: a flat ball on a chair (see ▶ Fig. 13.16), a double ball (see ▶ Fig. 13.2 and ▶ Fig. 13.3), a base that prevents the ball from rolling away (▶ Fig. 12.1), or no ball at all.
- When sitting on a ball, exercises can be done between two chairs, in a corner, or in front of a wall to prevent the ball from rolling away.

Exercise barefoot or wearing tennis shoes on a carpeted floor or nonslip mat.

- The ball needs to be clean and firm, with the correct amount of pressure according to the manufacturer's specifications.
- The size of the ball depends on the individual's size and mobility. The person seated on the ball should be able to maintain a good upright posture easily. Usually, this occurs when hips and knees are bent at no less than 90 degrees.
- Some exercises require two individuals sitting back to back on the same ball that must be large enough to accommodate two people (▶ Fig. 12.2).
- A resistive elastic band (TheraBand®) can be used to train the back extensors while exercising the pelvic floor muscles. This exercise is beneficial for preventing osteoporosis. The resistance of the band depends on the strength of the individual using it.

12.2 Positional Challenges to the Pelvic Girdle Organs

12.2.1 Prolapsed Uterus

Women with a prolapsed uterus or bladder may benefit from exercises which "unload" the pelvic floor (▶ Fig. 12.3, ▶ Fig. 12.4, ▶ Fig. 12.5, ▶ Fig. 12.6, ▶ Fig. 12.7, ▶ Fig. 12.8 and, ▶ Fig. 12.9).

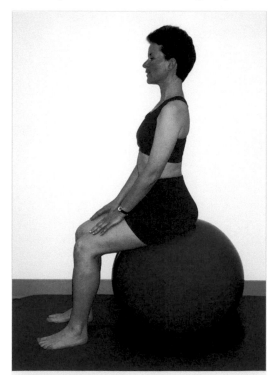

Fig. 12.1 A base under the ball prevents it from rolling away.

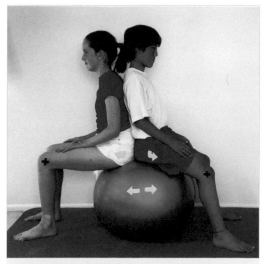

Fig. 12.2 Two individuals sharing one ball require a larger size ball.

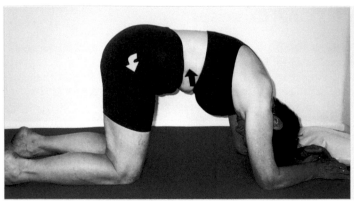

Fig. 12.3 The pelvic floor is "unloaded" in a low puppy position.

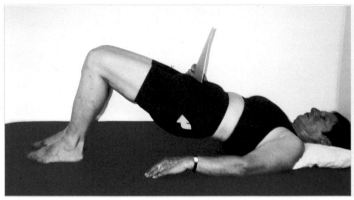

Fig. 12.4 Lifting the hips "unloads" the pelvic floor.

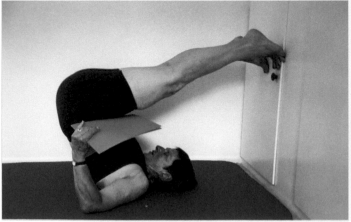

Fig. 12.5 A shoulder stand decreases the load on the pelvic floor.

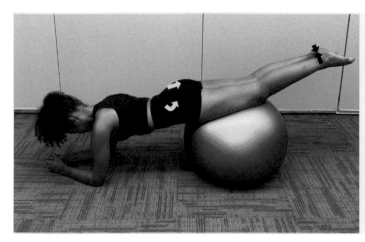

Fig. 12.6 Leaning forward, face down, over the ball may improve the topography of the uterus that is tilted backward (goldfish exercise).

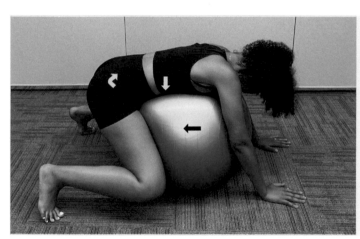

Fig. 12.7 Resting on a ball, face down, may improve the topography of the uterus that is tilted backward.

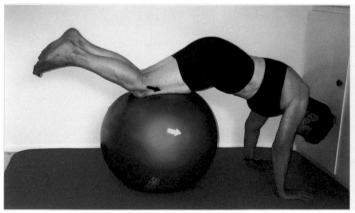

Fig. 12.8 Pulling the knees under the abdomen can coordinate with the tightening of the pelvic floor muscles.

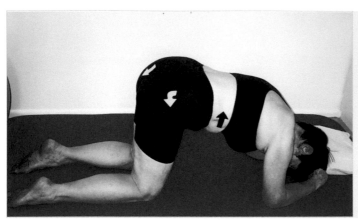

Fig. 12.9 Exhalation and tightening of the abdominal and pelvic floor muscles on "all fours" resting on the elbows.

The following example describes the feelings of a woman with severe incontinence problems following a prolapse of the uterus. At first, the doctor considered surgical repair, but after approximately 15 treatments, it was not necessary as the patient no longer felt the pressure from the prolapse. She no longer required medication for her urgencies, and her constipation was much improved.

Example

One patient's experience: "I had no more self-esteem. After the birth of my second child, the trouble began. At age 40, I had to go to the bathroom every 30 minutes during the day, and during sexual intercourse, I was leaking urine; it was embarrassing. I suffered from constipation and felt the pressure of the uterus bearing down into the vagina. Now, after several months of exercising, I only go to the bathroom about every 3 hours and no longer feel that I smell bad. My sex life is improved, and so is my self-esteem. Massaging my abdomen improved my constipation. The pressure of the uterus is gone."

Physical Therapy Treatment Options

- Review of anatomy and physiology (**see Part I**)
- Practice unloading the pelvic floor muscles (▶ Video 12.1 and ▶ Video 12.2)
- Breathing exercises

- Pelvic floor exercises in all planes, beginning in positions that decrease the load on the pelvic floor and progressing to sitting and standing
- Combination of breathing with pelvic floor exercises
- Training of daily activities without straining and with correct use of the pelvic floor muscles
- Colon massage, modalities, self-relaxation, soft-tissue mobilization, and acupuncture are additional treatment options
- Select positions for sexual intercourse that unload the pelvis

Suitable Exercises

Possible starting positions:
- On hands and knees with the forearms resting on the floor (▶ Fig. 12.3)
- On the back with the knees bent and hips lifted (▶ Fig. 12.4)
- Comfortable shoulder stand (▶ Fig. 12.5)
- Leaning over the ball with the head down and feet in the air (▶ Fig. 12.6)

In the illustrations, the cardboard indicates the position of the pelvic floor in space (▶ Fig. 12.4 and ▶ Fig. 12.5 and ▶ Video 12.3).

12.2.2 Backward-Tilting Uterus

In some women, the uterus is tilted backward. Exercises can help to improve the position of the uterus. Gravity and body weight can help to enhance the topography.

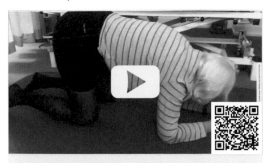

Video 12.1 Corrective exercise in quadruped position for prolapse with pelvic unloading

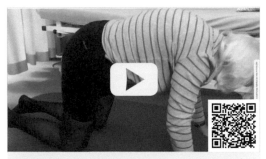

Video 12.2 Corrective exercise in quadruped position for prolapse with weight shift and hip rocking

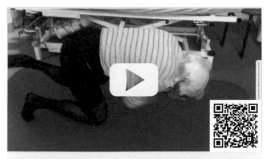

Video 12.3 Corrective exercise for pelvic unloading

Physical Therapy Treatment Options

- Review of anatomy and physiology (see **Part I**)
- Practice unloading the pelvic floor muscles with props (wedges, Swiss ball), bridging, and other exercises outlined in this book
- Practice finding positions that improve the topography of the uterus and encourage a forward position when indicated
- Breathing exercises
- Pelvic floor exercises in all planes, beginning in positions that decrease the load on the pelvic floor and improve the position of the uterus
- Combination of breathing with pelvic floor exercises
- Training of daily activities without straining and with correct use of the pelvic floor muscles

Suitable Exercises

- You may start on all fours or leaning over the ball, face down and feet in the air, or a low puppy position (► Fig. 12.6, ► Fig. 12.7, ► Fig. 12.8).

Pearl

- The pressure and compression of the ball in front of the pelvis in many cases can cause relief or proprioceptive awareness.
- More experienced individuals can try pulling the knees below the stomach (► Fig. 12.8).

Note

- As soon as possible, one should progress to sitting and standing positions, because these positions are most functional. These positions put the pelvic floor in a more horizontal position relative to gravity and support the weight of the inner organs (such as the bladder, uterus, and rectum).
- Exercises should always include training of fast- and slow-twitch muscle fibers.
- Exercises should provoke contractions of the muscle fibers in different planes.
- All of the above exercises are appropriate for men and children who suffer from pelvic floor weakness.
- Colon massage, modalities, self-relaxation, soft-tissue mobilization, and acupuncture are additional treatment options.

12.3 Prostate Surgery

Many men scheduled for prostate surgery are unaware of what to expect from the procedure or what to expect following the surgery. Surgery that does not remove the prostate gland does not necessarily result in incontinence, but it can. Following a radical prostatectomy (removal of the prostate gland), some men experience temporary incontinence. Their recovery can also be impacted by the method of prostate removal, the number of port sites, robotic or standard surgery and if the nerves are spared in the procedure. Procedures for prostate removal necessitate the use of a catheter during the initial healing phase which lasts from 1 to 3 weeks. After removal of the catheter, temporary incontinence is normal but should be resolved within 6 to 8 weeks. In some cases, this incontinence does not get resolved and can last up to 12 months. These patients can still recover their continence. A small percentage of men may be permanently incontinent.[58] Very few men know that they have an internal sphincter muscle of the bladder, which is not under voluntary control and is a passive control mechanism for continence. The internal (proximal) sphincter muscle consists of a layer of mucosal tissue with a high amount of blood vessels, smooth muscles, and elastic fibers.

The sympathetic nervous system innervates the sphincter muscle. During surgery, this internal sphincter can be damaged, resulting in a patient's dependence on the external sphincter muscles to be continent. The external sphincter (or rhabdosphincter) muscle is under voluntary control. It has two layers of skeletal muscles that are supplied by the pudendal nerve, which also innervates the pelvic floor muscles. Some fibers of its inner layer are connected with the urethra. As a result, these muscles maintain their resting muscle tone and do not fatigue. These fibers are under autonomic control and contribute to passive continence.[3]

The continence mechanism in men from the internal sphincter to the external sphincter is continuous as the fibers from the internal sphincter interweave with those of the external sphincter.[17,18] Understanding how to contract the pelvic floor muscles and the external sphincter of the urethra, and how to include the contraction into daily activities, can prepare the patient for potentially reduced control of the internal sphincter after surgery and the subsequent continence challenges. All exercises should be coordinated with breathing to decrease strain on the pelvic floor. Correct breathing mechanics is essential to establish the most optimal environment for training the pelvic floor. Initiating breath work early on in the recovery establishes patterns that can be built upon while patient regains their function and activities of daily living.

> **Pearl**
>
> It is much easier to learn and practice the relevant exercises (e.g., lifting objects) before surgery than afterward.

Two sessions before surgery should suffice as an introduction to learning the exercises, understanding the functions of the internal and external sphincter muscles of the urethra, and learning correct breathing and lifting. The second session should allow the patient to review the exercises and ask questions.

In a study conducted at Kaiser Foundation Hospital in Los Angeles, 66% of postradical prostatectomy patients were continent at 16 weeks after surgery.[22] Those patients who were treated to two exercise sessions before surgery regained continence earlier than the control group.

12.3.1 Physical Therapy Treatment Options

- Review of anatomy and physiology (**see Part I**)
- Breathing exercises
- Pelvic floor exercises in all planes
- Combination of breathing with pelvic floor exercises
- Training of daily activities without straining and with correct use of the pelvic floor muscles (▶ Video 12.4, ▶ Video 12.5, ▶ Video 12.6, ▶ Video 12.7, ▶ Video 12.8, ▶ Video 12.9, ▶ Video 12.10, and ▶ Video 12.11).

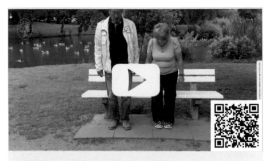

Video 12.4 Corrective functional movements with slow fiber activation while sitting down

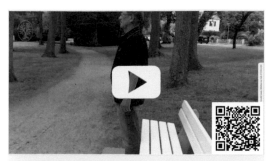

Video 12.5 Corrective functional movements with slow fiber activation through standing and sitting—side view

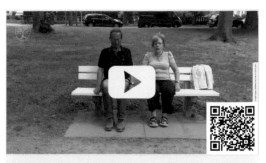

Video 12.6 Corrective functional movements with fast fiber activation—connect and go

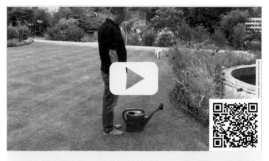

Video 12.7 Corrective functional movements with slow fiber activation—shoe tying

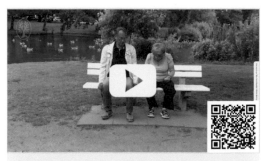

Video 12.8 Corrective activation of fast fiber through sitting and standing

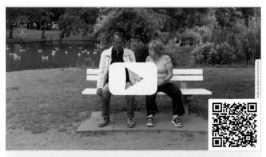

Video 12.9 Corrective training in bending—slow fiber activation

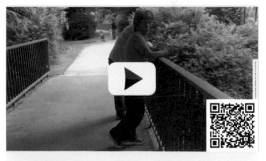

Video 12.10 Corrective training in fast standing from sitting position—slow and fast fiber

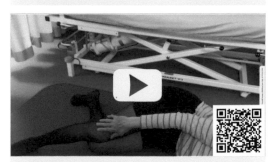

Video 12.11 Prolapse correction in sidelying position

12.3.2 Suitable Exercises Before Prostate Surgery

Before prostate surgery, the patient may benefit from learning how to breathe correctly to avoid straining and bearing down on the pelvic floor in all daily activities. Even though the patient may not be allowed to lift heavy objects right after surgery, it is crucial to practice proper lifting before surgery.

- After learning to contract the anal sphincter in isolation, the patient can practice contracting the muscles (ischiocavernosus, bulbocavernosus) in front of the looks ok toilette seat by pretending to squirt out the last drop of urine. This contraction is felt at the base of the penis. The patient can also practice the coordination of muscle activation with exhalation.

- When lying on the belly, the patient can try to contract the anal sphincter in isolation, then contract the buttock muscles also, and finally, to relax the buttock muscles while keeping the anus puckered (▶ Fig. 12.10).
- A pillow should be placed under the abdomen to avoid back pain and increase the mobility of pelvis and hips.
- Exercises without a ball can be done lying on the back or side and on the hands and knees.
- Lying on the back, exhalation is coordinated with puckering the anus and lifting the pelvis off the ground (▶ Fig. 12.11).
- On the hands and knees and in a side-lying position, the pelvis is tilted backward during exhalation and slightly forward during inhalation (▶ Fig. 12.12, ▶ Fig. 12.13, ▶ Fig. 12.14).

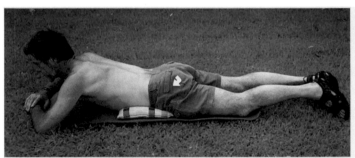

Fig. 12.10 Contracting the pelvic floor muscles while lying on the stomach.

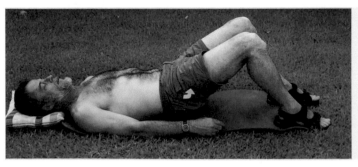

Fig. 12.11 The pelvic floor muscles are activated during exhalation when lying on the back.

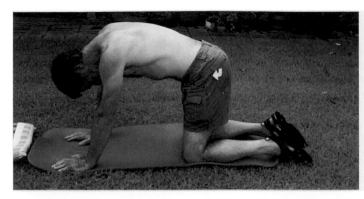

Fig. 12.12 On the hands and knees, the pelvis can be tilted in a backward direction during exhalation.

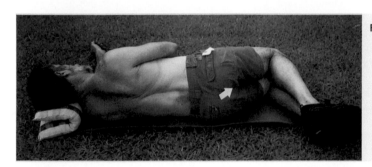

Fig. 12.13 Side-lying exhalation.

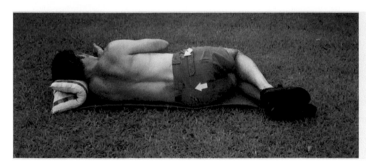

Fig. 12.14 Side-lying inhalation.

- As proper lifting requires a wide base of support, the low back muscles must be in a neutral position. This position ensures optimal muscle recruitment and biomechanical balance of all of the structures involved with proper and effective stabilization of the lumbar spine.
- The pelvic floor muscles should contract during exhalation.
- It is important to avoid straining the pelvic floor muscles or increasing abdominal pressure (Valsalva maneuver) during lifting (► Fig. 12.15 and ► Fig. 12.16).
- All of the exercises described in this book for training awareness and strength of the pelvic floor muscles in all directions and planes can be practiced before surgery.
- Favorite activities from a patient's exercise program can be reviewed and adapted to include strengthening of the pelvic floor muscles to avoid straining while exercising.
- Many men prefer to use a Swiss ball for the exercises for the comfort of the prostate gland.
- Patients should practice urinating in sitting position as this allows the urethra to be in a straight position and the urine to flow better.[3] Urinating in sitting position may also prevent high residuals of urine in the bladder.
- Contraction of the pelvic floor muscles before coughing and sneezing can be practiced before surgery.

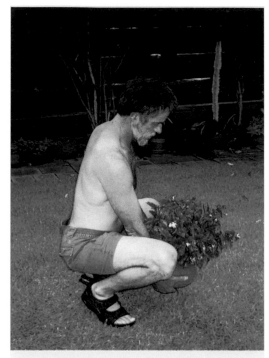

Fig. 12.15 Starting position when lifting a heavy object.

12.3.3 Suitable Exercises after Prostate Surgery

After surgery, the patient usually wears a catheter. Depending on the reason for surgery, the patient's overall health and condition, and the seriousness of the operation, the patient's condition afterward can vary considerably.

- Exercises begin with the coordination of breathing and gentle puckering of the anal sphincter, especially before coughing and sneezing. It is equally important for men to exercise the muscles in the front (bulbocavernosus and ischiocavernosus) by

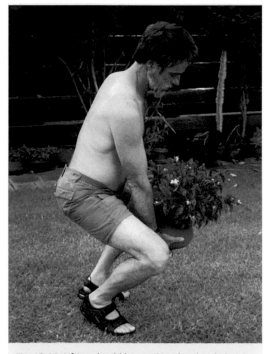

Fig. 12.16 Lifting should be combined with exhalation while tightening the pelvic floor and abdominal muscles.

pretending to squirt out the last drop of urine and feel a scrotal lift.

- Once the catheter is removed, and the doctor has approved further exercises, a therapist should reevaluate the patient's condition and review exercises according to the findings.
- Usually, pelvic floor contraction can be intensified after the catheter is removed. Precontractions are recommended before turning in bed, changing from lying to a seated position, and from a sitting to a standing position.
- Before the patient begins to drive again, these precontractions should also be practiced when moving the legs into and out of a car.
- The exercises described above (▶ Fig. 12.3, ▶ Fig. 12.4, and ▶ Fig. 12.11, ▶ Fig. 12.12, ▶ Fig. 12.13, ▶ Fig. 12.14) should be done, adjusting the intensity so as not to increase the pain.
- The progression of exercises depends on the speed and extent of the patient's recovery and the doctor's findings. The patient can always contact the surgeon with any questions about the progress. The therapist should adapt the exercises to the individual's needs.
- When sitting on the ball, the exercises should primarily be performed in a forward/backward direction to avoid straining the scar until it is well healed. Healing may take about 4 to 6 weeks.
- The patient then slowly progresses with Swiss ball exercises in all directions and increases the contraction around the urethra (in front of the seat, near the base of the penis).
- After a prostatectomy, bladder dysfunction and inability to tighten the external sphincter of the urethra can cause incontinence. Other individuals may suffer from urine retention, which may cause overflow and dribbling.[70]
- Incontinence can occur after prostate surgery for benign hyperplasia of the prostate.
- All clients have to develop a keen awareness of when they are leaking urine. The therapist can customize the exercises for individual clients. The activity that is causing leakage can be

practiced by taking the movement sequence as a whole apart and training only individual movement sequences at first.

- Slow fibers of the pelvic floor are trained by holding a contraction for 5 to 10 seconds or more; fast fibers are trained with repeated quick contractions (quick flicks). Both muscle fiber types of the pelvic floor muscles should be trained.

Pearl

- Most clients, after radical prostatectomy, are much improved at 4 to 12 weeks after surgery; a small number may leak urine for up to a year, and an even smaller percentage can leak beyond this time frame.
- Patients who have problems with erections after surgery need to discuss this with the surgeon. If the nerve is preserved during radical prostatectomy, the patient's erectile function may improve with exercises, erection aids, medication, or a combination of these.[17]
- Biofeedback, electrical stimulation, self-relaxation, and other treatments, including medication, may be required if leakage of urine persists. Close cooperation among the doctor, therapist, and patient is required.

Example 1

Months after a radical prostatectomy, a patient came to therapy because he was still leaking urine and had to wear several pads a day. When he reported leakage, especially when getting in and out of the car, the exercises described in Chapter 13 and ▶ Fig. 11.5 and ▶ Fig. 11.6, were prescribed. Lying on his back with the feet on the ball, he learned to precontract the pelvic floor muscles before moving the legs on a stable body. The patient then learned to coordinate the movements in a sitting position when getting out of the car, and the leakage decreased.

Example 2

At another treatment session, the same client explained that he was leaking, especially after going to the bathroom and when relaxing: "Yesterday I did great, I did not leak at all for most of the day." When asked what he had done the day before, he answered, "I had to go to a funeral and then go shopping. Then I went to the bathroom, and after that, I started leaking again." The client probably did well because his attention and muscle tone increased during the activities of the morning. He was instructed to practice puckering at least 10 times immediately after emptying the bladder and eliminating his bowels, holding each contraction for up to 10 seconds. To increase the resting tone of the pelvic floor muscles, the client was also instructed to pretend to hold a lentil with the anal sphincter at all times. These instructions helped the client to improve his continence further.

12.4 Pain of the Pelvic Floor Muscles and Leakage of Urine during Intercourse

There are many reasons for pain and discomfort during sexual intercourse (dyspareunia). Studies have shown that 20 to 40% of women affected by dyspareunia were sexually abused or raped before the age of 18 years, and 10 to 25% of the married women questioned reported sexual violence by their husbands at some time in their marriage.[66] Instead of talking to a doctor or therapist, these victims often suffer silently and can have many problems. These issues may include pain, incontinence of stool (fecal incontinence) or urine, constipation, and other gastrointestinal symptoms (stomach and bowel problems).

Leakage of urine during sexual intercourse is a problem affecting the self-esteem of many women. In addition to incontinence and diseases, prolapse (see Prolapsed Uterus or Bladder [p. 47]) can cause pain and leakage of urine during sexual intercourse. The problem can also stem from a difficult birth or other injuries and scars in the pelvis or pelvic floor area.

Again, many individuals suffer in silence because they are not aware that, in most cases, this is a treatable condition. The first step, therefore, is a thorough evaluation by a doctor who can determine which other treatments are indicated. Supportive treatment by a psychologist can take place parallel to physical therapy treatment.

12.4.1 Physical Therapy Treatment Options

- Review of anatomy and physiology (see **Part I**)
- Breathing exercises (see Chapter 9 [p. 29])
- Pelvic floor exercises in all planes
- Combination of breathing with pelvic floor exercises; emphasis on relaxation if the pelvic floor is tight (see Chapter 7 [p. 23]) and on strengthening exercises if the pelvic floor muscles are weak
- Connective-tissue massage
- Manual therapy
- Visceral mobilization
- Colon massage
- Treatment of scar tissue
- Biofeedback
- Electrical stimulation
- Acupuncture
- Heat or cold treatment

Note

- Evaluation and treatment of the area surrounding the pelvic floor (bony structure of the pelvis, viscera, hips, low back) may be required.
- Treatment of constipation to avoid straining and stretching of the pelvic floor muscles is especially indicated in patients who leak urine and patients with a prolapse.
- The exercises should improve the sensory awareness of the pelvic floor and enable the individual to relax during penetration and be able to contract the pelvic floor muscles around the penis. It is important to be in control of the pelvic floor and understand its function.
- Vaginal weights (cones) may be beneficial to some patients, but there is always the possibility that the training is not done correctly, nor can it be considered a very functional training. In some patients, it is useful as a progression.

Example

A woman in her early forties came to physical therapy because of chronic low back pain. Past treatments had been unsuccessful. During the evaluation, there were indications of a possible history of sexual abuse. For example, early menopause, insecure behavior, back pain which did not respond to treatment, and connective-tissue zone at the low back. This zone symptom is common in women who suffer from infrequent menstruation (oligomenorrhea). When questioned about a history of possible sexual abuse, the client stated that she had been abused 10 years previously. The possible correlation between the back pain and the abuse was explained, pointing out that the brain does not forget events easily.

Treatment began with connective-tissue massage of the low back and the sacral area before the patient was introduced to pelvic floor exercises. The patient was also given heat treatments for the back and had the opportunity to talk about personal issues. She was encouraged to have counseling by a psychologist or psychiatrist. Pelvic floor exercises for sensory awareness and activities with and without a ball, as described in this book, combined with breathing exercises, helped this woman to become free of pain.

An example of a woman who was leaking urine during sexual intercourse is provided in Chapter 12, Prolapsed or Backward-Tilting Uterus (p. 50). Usually, emphasis should be on strengthening the pelvic floor muscles and increasing sensory awareness. Scars in the area of the pelvic floor and the abdominal compartment deserve special attention and treatment. A thorough evaluation precedes physical therapy treatment.

12.5 Injuries to the Pelvic Region following Accidents

Sometimes it is difficult to find a doctor who understands the many symptoms a person can suffer from an injury that affects the autonomic nervous system.[75] An accident can cause pelvic pain, incontinence, urgencies, and other symptoms, especially diffuse pain. For example, a fall onto the sacrum or tail bone can cause problems of the pelvic floor because the pudendal nerve and the parasympathetic nerves (of the autonomic nervous system) leave the spinal canal at that level. The sympathetic nerves of the autonomic nervous system leave the spinal canal at the level of the lower thoracic spine.

These nerves can inhibit or stimulate the bladder and pelvic floor muscles and make the complicated pelvic floor a wonder of interactions, many of which are not yet fully understood. The pudendal nerve supplies the muscles of the pelvic floor (see ▶ Fig. 2.4).

A fall can cause injuries to the nerves as they exit the spinal canal and can also affect the bony integrity of the pelvis. Muscles and tendons can be pulled or damaged, and all structures involved deserve treatment. A difficult birth can cause similar injuries to those same structures and nerves. Therefore, many of the symptoms are possible after a complicated delivery or prolonged labor.

12.5.1 Physical Therapy Treatment Options

In addition to pelvic floor exercises, indicated for the treatment of incontinence of urine or stool, the following may be required:
- Review of anatomy and physiology and the autonomic nervous system (see **Part I**)
- Breathing exercises (see Chapter 11 [p. 42])
- Manual therapy
- Connective-tissue massage
- Nerve tissue mobilization
- Visceral mobilization
- Colon massage
- Modalities such as biofeedback, electrical stimulation, ultrasound, heat, or cold applications
- Acupuncture

The following examples will illustrate the complexity of pelvic pain problems.

Example 1

A healthy young man did a cannonball jump into a swimming pool. For 4 years, he saw many doctors for the following complaints: frequency of urination, prostate pain, inflammation of the prostate (prostatitis), scrotal pain, premature ejaculations (all probably related to parasympathetic nerve injury), and coccygodynia (pain in the tail bone region). The patient also complained about pelvic pain and the inability to sit. This most probably was related to the jolt sustained by the bony structure of the pelvis when hitting the water. Medications, including antibiotics, were tried but did not help. Some of the complaints resolved or diminished over time.

The client appeared to have hit the water hard, landing on the sacrum, which had probably caused damage to the nerves of the autonomic nervous system and dysbalance of the bony structures of the pelvis. Therapy was directed at the sacral area where the soft tissue was very tight and required mobilization. Therapy goals, therefore, included restoring mobility of the soft tissue at the sacrum, the lumbar spine, and the pelvis. Strengthening the pelvic floor and surrounding muscles also formed part of the treatment. Manual therapy was selected to improve the balance of the pelvic girdle.[12]

All treatments led to a significant improvement in the client's condition. Tight muscles were stretched to improve the ability to effortlessly maintain good posture when sitting and standing.

Example 2

A 40-year-old woman fell from a horse, getting one leg caught in the stirrup. As she fell, her legs were pulled apart, and one side of the sacrum and buttock hit the ground. She came to therapy for hip pain and separation of the symphysis pubis.

After the accident, the client described clitoral pain ("I thought this was from riding the horse"), frequent urination, and pelvic floor pain in the center of the seat and at the tail bone (coccygodynia). Her leg muscles, especially of the inner thigh of her left leg (adductor muscles), were excruciating. She needed crutches for walking even short distances.

Treatment began with her back to loosen up the tight connective tissue of the sacral area. (If the patient had come immediately after the injury, manual lymph drainage treatment would have been another option.) In addition to stretching the adductor muscle and its associated nerves (which can refer pain right into the center of the seat[69]), she may have stretched the nerves that innervate the pelvic floor, the clitoris, and the bladder. The client's condition significantly improved once the cause of the pain was understood, and treatment directed toward the injured areas.

During the second phase of the treatment, biofeedback was added because the client could not relax her pelvic floor muscles. Using visualization and auditory feedback improved her awareness of her pelvic floor muscles.

Kinesiotaping (using Japanese elastic tape) was used to support the muscle function and stabilize the hip. Ice and heat applications were used at home to manage the pain. The patient continued to improve and was able to return to work and walk without assistive devices.

12.6 Incontinence of Gas (Flatulence), Fecal Incontinence, and Hemorrhoids

Evaluation should include the abdominal compartment and eating and drinking habits. Nutritional counseling is often indicated. The client must develop good toilet and nutritional habits (see Chapters 6 and 7) as part of the treatment. Developing sensory awareness of the pelvic floor and understanding the process of bowel elimination are imperative for success.

Many individuals suffer from both anal and urinary incontinence and hemorrhoids. Some patients are unable to grade their contraction of the anal sphincter and the vagina. Practice can include pretending to hold objects of different weights (e.g., lentils, marbles, cherries) or contracting the pelvic floor muscles upward and inward like an elevator moving up to the third floor. Such exercises can help to achieve a graded contraction and relaxation. After learning to pucker the anal sphincter muscles, coordination of breathing and contraction of the anus during exhalation follows.

The client can then practice various ball exercises, but should not forget to lift correctly without exerting increased pressure to the pelvic floor muscles (Valsalva maneuver) (see ▶ Fig. 12.10 and ▶ Fig. 12.11. See also ▶ Video 12.13 and ▶ Video 12.14). Proper postural alignment is essential and should be achieved without difficulty; it may require stretching tight muscles surrounding the pelvis.

Constipation is part of the problem and can be treated with colon massage,[33] connective-tissue massage,[61] and visceral mobilization (▶ Video 12.12, ▶ Video 12.13, ▶ Video 12.14, and ▶ Video 12.15).

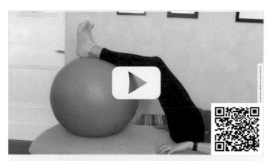

Video 12.12 Flatus correction through abduction in sidelying position

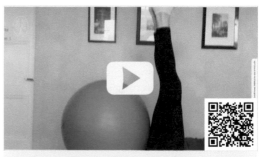

Video 12.13 Postpartum flatus correction with Swiss ball—bilateral hip abduction

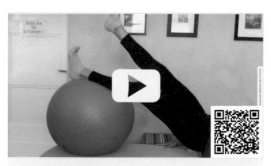

Video 12.14 Postpartum flatus correction with Swiss ball—single leg bridge

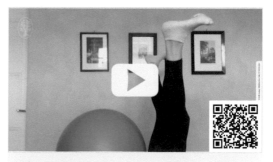

Video 12.15 Flatus correction in sidelying position

12.6.1 Physical Therapy Treatment Options

- Review of anatomy and physiology (see **Part I**)
- Breathing exercises
- Sensory awareness training of the anal sphincter
- Pelvic floor exercises
- Combination of breathing with pelvic floor exercises emphasizing relaxation if the pelvic floor is tight and strengthening if the pelvic floor muscle is weak
- Connective-tissue massage
- Manual therapy
- Visceral mobilization
- Colon massage
- Treatment of scar tissue
- Biofeedback
- Electrical stimulation

Example

A 69-year-old, very motivated client came to therapy for the treatment of fecal incontinence that had begun 4 years earlier. The client had no awareness of when she was losing stool. She also suffered from an inability to control gas and from urinary incontinence. The client had a good understanding of the anatomy but poor awareness of her anal sphincter and levator ani muscles.

Kegel exercises[36] performed in previous therapy sessions did not help the patient. She was given sensory awareness training of the pelvic floor muscles, especially of the anal sphincter muscle. She was also given gentle abdominal treatment and instructed to self-massage her abdomen, which was very tight but relaxed with treatment. The very motivated client exercised at home and reported that she was continent within weeks after the first instruction.

12.7 Treatment of Children with Incontinence

Children must understand that they have muscles under their control, which can help them stay dry at night. The concept that the bladder is a storage area for urine is essential as well. Once I was shown pictures drawn by children with incontinence. They had been asked where urine came from, and their drawings depicted a straight line from the mouth to the genitals with no bladder (place to store urine). Using illustrations or a water-filled balloon, children can learn the concept of storing the urine and emptying the bladder. For example, keeping the opening closed to keep the water in the balloon or relaxing the opening and allowing the balloon to empty, just as the bladder would function.

Children need to be motivated, and it may be useful to let them name the exercises, writing them down, and mark how often and when they practice them. Sometimes it helps to mark a voiding diary in different colors or let the children report to the therapist (rather than the parents) when they practice the exercises. Children can have many problems, both with leakage and retention of urine, and each child requires very individual attention.[72]

Most exercises in this book are appropriate for children. The Swiss ball is a very motivating tool for the children to exercise with.

Note

- Children are not small adults; their attention span, motivation, and judgment differ from adults.
- For safety, adjust exercises to the child's ability and supervise the child until he or she masters the task.
- Do not let children exercise unsupervised with the elastic band.
- Exercising before going to sleep may have a carry-over effect and promote dryness.
- When sitting on the toilet, children need to have their feet supported, for example, on a stool.

12.7.1 Physical Therapy Treatment Options

- Review of anatomy and physiology, making the child understand how the muscles of the bladder and the pelvic floor work together
- Breathing exercises
- Pelvic floor exercises

- Combination of breathing with pelvic floor exercises
- Biofeedback
- Electrical stimulation
- Occasionally, the following treatment options may also be helpful:
  - Connective-tissue massage
  - Manual therapy
  - Visceral mobilization
  - Colon massage
  - Treatment of scar tissue

Example

One of the children in this book suffered from frequent bed-wetting and became continent when practicing to be a "movie star" in the video. The child had received various recommended therapies, none of which helped. The fun exercises with the Swiss ball appeared to be the motivating factor.

13 Functional Exercises for the Pelvic Floor

13.1 Exercises with the Swiss Ball

Once the therapist and client have familiarized themselves with the practical exercises, many other activities are adaptable for functional strengthening of the pelvic floor muscles. Exercising with the ball is also beneficial to improving pelvic floor muscle strength, in that the muscles surrounding the pelvic floor are strengthened as well.

A client over 70 years old recently reported that after 3 months' training, she had fewer problems getting up from the floor and felt her strength had improved. She told the following story:

Example

"When I first came to learn pelvic floor exercises because of leakage of urine, my 3-year-old grandson had pointed to my belly saying 'grandma baby!' Approximately 3 months later, my grandson pointed to my belly, saying 'grandma no baby!' He had discovered that my belly had gotten a lot flatter. The exercises helped me, not only for the pelvic floor but also to increase the strength in my legs and to flatten my protruding abdomen. I feel good and enjoy exercising now, the other day I practiced while waiting in a car, to the rhythm of music."

Because most people spend a fair amount of time in bed, it is also recommended to learn exercises that can be done lying on the back or the side. Exercising before sleeping or getting up in the morning increases sensory awareness of individuals who have problems with incontinence at night or before getting up in the morning. Children who wet the bed may also benefit from exercising the pelvic floor muscles before sleeping.

13.1.1 Lying on the Back with the Legs Bent

This position decreases the load on the pelvic floor because the pelvic floor muscles are mostly in a vertical position in space.

- First, breathe in and then breathe out, feeling the stomach rise and fall (see ▶ Fig. 11.1 and ▶ Fig. 11.2).
- Consciously relax the pelvic floor muscles during inhalation and arch the back slightly. Exhale and contract the pelvic floor muscles by puckering the anus and visualizing picking up a raisin through tightening of the vagina and urethra. The back flattens, and the pelvis does a little "sit up," that is, it tilts backward. For the slow muscle fibers, the contraction is held in this position for 5 to 10 seconds; for the fast-twitch fibers, the contractions are fast and repeated 5 to 10 times in quick succession (▶ Fig. 13.1). The intensity of the contractions is more important than repetitions.
- The same exercise can be done with a ball under the feet or on a double ball. Breathe in and arch the back, relax the pelvic floor, then exhale and

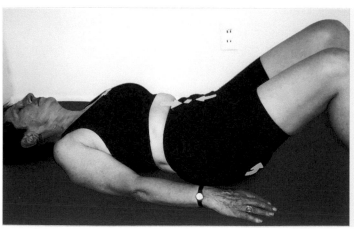

Fig. 13.1 Lying on the back, the pelvis is tilted backward, and the back flattened during exhalation. Exercises for slow and fast fibers can be done in this position.

push the legs away. The ball is pushed away, and the pelvis lifted while puckering and tightening the pelvic floor muscles. The buttock muscles are then also tightened (▶ Fig. 13.2 and ▶ Fig. 13.3).

• During exhalation, the ball can be lifted and moved toward the chest. This movement strengthens the abdominal and hamstring muscles (▶ Fig. 13.4; ▶ Video 13.1).

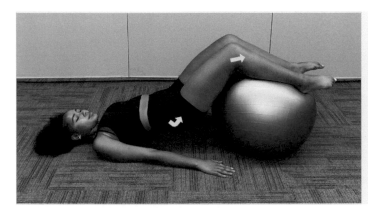

Fig. 13.2 Lying on the back, the ball is pushed away with the legs. The double ball provides greater stability than one ball.

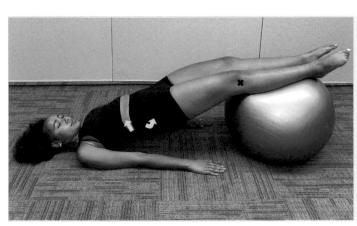

Fig. 13.3 To increase the degree of difficulty, the hips lift off the ground during exhalation.

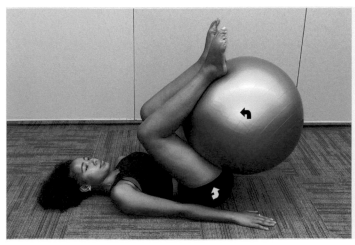

Fig. 13.4 Lifting the ball with the legs strengthens the hamstrings and abdominal muscles. The pelvic floor integrates these groups with this type of activity.

The pelvic floor muscles are integrated by puckering and tightening during exhalation.

- The direction of movement can be reversed: during inhalation, extend the legs on the ball and during exhalation flex the legs on the ball, which rolls toward the buttock. (This exercise is called "ball roll.")

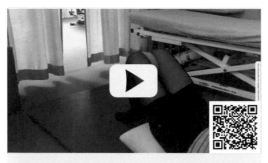

Video 13.1 Corrective pelvic floor unloading with Swiss ball squeeze in supine position

Note

- This exercise can be modified to practice leg movements on a stable trunk (e.g., similar to lifting the legs when getting out of a car). With the legs resting on the ball, move the legs from side to side after puckering and tightening the pelvic floor muscles. Relax the muscles after returning to the starting position (▶ Fig. 13.5 and ▶ Fig. 13.6).
- Lying on the back with a resistive elastic band (TheraBand) tied around the knees, the legs are spread against the resistance of the band during exhalation. This movement strengthens the abductor and external rotator muscles of the hips and relaxes the adductor and internal rotator muscles. When puckering at the same time, the pelvic floor muscles are strengthened.

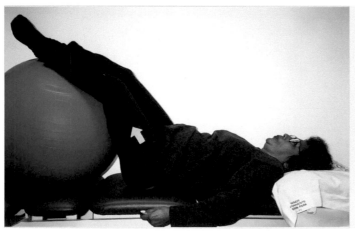

Fig. 13.5 Starting position for moving the legs to the side on a stable trunk.

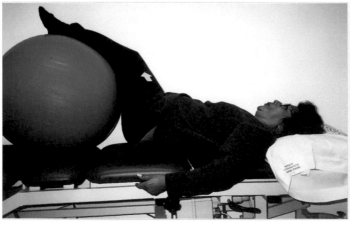

Fig. 13.6 This position is similar to lifting the legs out of a car and can be coordinated with breathing.

13.1.2 Lying on the Abdomen (Prone) Over the Ball

Lying prone over the ball is a favorite position for individuals with back discomfort. The abdomen is supported, and the exercises appear to relax the low back. The legs and arms should rest on the floor, either at the same time or alternately.

When lying on the abdomen on a mat, a pillow should be placed under the stomach to avoid back pain (see ▶ Fig. 12.10).

- Lying face down and resting over the ball, the back arches slightly during inhalation. During exhalation, the pelvic floor tightens, and the legs lifted. This movement strengthens the leg and back muscles (see ▶ Fig. 12.6, "goldfish" exercise).

- Land alternately on the feet and hands by rolling the ball forward and backward. During inhalation, the pelvic floor is relaxed and arched; during exhalation, the tail bone is pulled toward the pubic bone (▶ Fig. 13.7 and ▶ Fig. 13.8, "swing" exercise).

> **Note**
>
> - The contraction of the pelvic floor muscles is held for 5 to 10 seconds at the end of the movement.
> - As a progression, the exercises "goldfish" and "sea urchin"[14] can be adapted to train the pelvic floor.

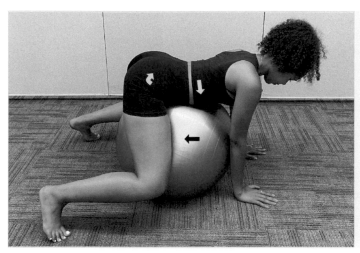

Fig. 13.7 Inhalation against the ball; the pelvis is tilted forward, the back arched.

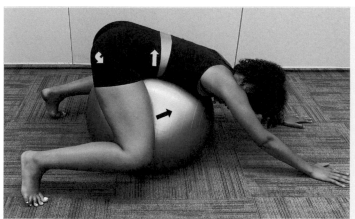

Fig. 13.8 During exhalation, the tail bone is pulled toward the pubic bone. The lumbar spine flattens.

13.1.3 Sitting on the Ball

Since many people spend a great deal of time sitting, functional exercises should also be practiced in a sitting position.

- Train sensory awareness by puckering and contracting the anal sphincter, urethra, and/ or vagina.
- Possible progressions include adding movements of the ball in all directions as well as bouncing on the ball. The pelvic floor muscles are in a horizontal position in space; they have to carry the load of the viscera (the organs within the pelvis).

Note

- In the sitting position, all movements initiate from the sitting bones; neither chest nor knees move in space.
- With all the exercises, the fast fibers are trained by quickly repeating contractions (quick flicks) while the slow fibers are trained by holding the contraction for 5 to 10 seconds at the end of the movement.
- All movements can and should be coordinated with breathing. The pelvic floor muscles relax during inhalation and contract during exhalation.

Possible Progression of Exercises

- Select the right ball. Good upright sitting posture happens when the hips are positioned slightly higher than the knees.
- Use a double ball or a flat ball if this improves safety.
- Choose a safe environment. First, practice between two chairs or hold onto something fixed until you feel safe enough to do the exercises without support.
- Learn the exercise first without thinking about the pelvic floor, just feel the movement.
- Limit the movement to the pelvis by keeping the knees and chest still. When the sitting bones move the ball, the pelvic floor muscles are involved. By puckering the anus and tightening the urethra (in women also the vagina) during exhalation, the contraction intensifies.
- Remember to train both fast and slow fibers of the pelvic floor muscles by quickly repeating the contractions and holding them to a count of 5 to 10.

- Add forced exhalation by making a guttural sound, similar to static on the radio, in the back of the throat while tightening the pelvic floor. One could pretend to cough or sneeze, or say words such as "kick" or "cool" (▶ Fig. 13.8).
- Add bouncing movements. Chose a safe place, such as a corner of the room, where the ball cannot roll away.
- Say explosive words such as "kick" or "cool" while bouncing.
- Bounce more forcefully, swinging the arms forward and upward. Make fists when contracting the pelvic floor muscles and open the hands when relaxing them.

13.1.4 Rolling the Ball Forward and Backward and Side to Side

- Keep knees and chest still while the sitting bones "grip" the ball, rolling it forward during exhalation. Hold the contraction, then relax and let the ball roll backward.
- Moving the ball in a forward/backward direction (▶ Fig. 13.9) trains the fibers of the levator ani muscle, which runs from the pubic bone to the tail bone.

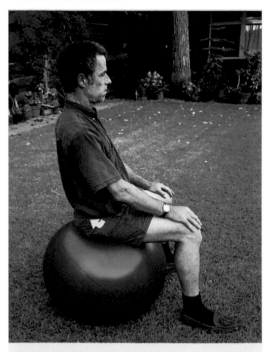

Fig. 13.9 The ball is rolled backward, and the pelvic floor relaxed during inhalation. The ball is gripped with the sitting bones while moving forward.

- Tightening the anal sphincter before moving the ball from the center to one side trains those fibers that run from one side to the other (▶ Fig. 13.10, ▶ Video 13.2).
- Lean forward against a wall with the hands and knees touching the wall. This action helps to learn to restrict the movement of the pelvis to only forward/backward, side to side, or diagonally (▶ Fig. 13.11 and ▶ Fig. 13.12, see also ▶ Video 13.3 and ▶ Video 13.4).

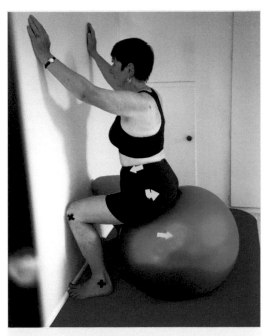

Fig. 13.11 Leaning against a wall with the knees and hands limits the movement of the chest and knees. The sitting bones move the ball.

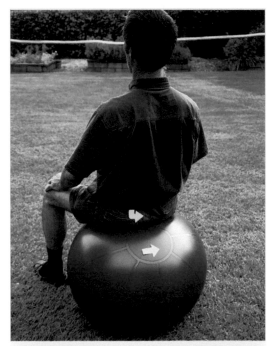

Fig. 13.10 The ball can be rolled from side to side. One sitting bone grips the ball and moves it. At the end of the movement, the position is held for 5 to 10 seconds before relaxing.

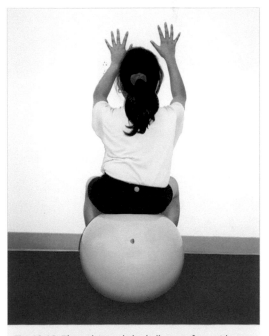

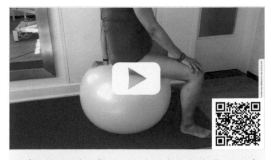

Video 13.2 Pelvic floor stretch with Swiss ball—seated diagonal movements

Fig. 13.12 The pelvis and the ball move from side to side.

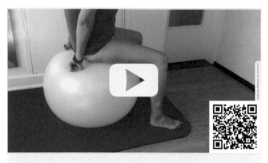

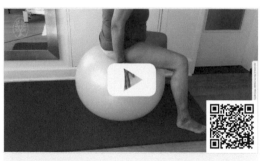

Video 13.3 Pelvic floor stretch with Swiss ball—seated sagittal movements

Video 13.4 Pelvic floor stretch with Swiss ball—seated lateral movements

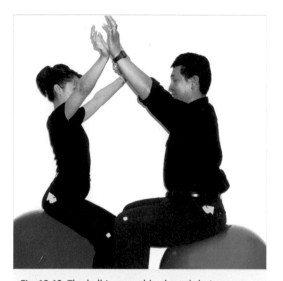

Fig. 13.13 The ball is moved backward during inhalation.

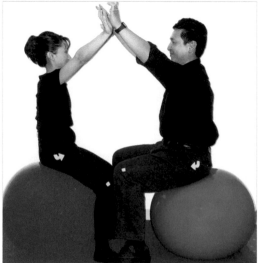

Fig. 13.14 The sitting bones move the ball forward during exhalation. Hands and knees do not move in space.

- Movement of the knees and trunk can also be restricted if two individuals face each other with their hands and their knees touching (▶ Fig. 13.13 and ▶ Fig. 13.14).

13.1.5 Rolling the Ball in a Diagonal Direction

The ball is an excellent tool for moving the pelvis in all directions. Some of the muscle fibers of the levator ani muscle and the outer layer of the pelvic floor (urogenital diaphragm) run in a diagonal direction. Muscles can strengthen best with exercises that shorten muscles in the direction of the muscle fibers. The contractions can be fast or slow

and held at the end of the movement. Relax the pelvic floor during inhalation and backward movement.

- Start as described above (▶ Fig. 13.9, ▶ Fig. 13.10, ▶ Fig. 13.11, ▶ Fig. 13.12, ▶ Fig. 13.13, ▶ Fig. 13.14), but this time move the left sitting bone in the direction of the right knee. As always, the knees and chest do not move. All the movement comes from the pelvis.
- The above exercises are done with resistance by pushing the ball in the opposite direction of the movement of the pelvis (▶ Fig. 13.15).
- The exercise can be done on the ball "cushion" if it cannot be done safely on a ball (▶ Fig. 13.16).

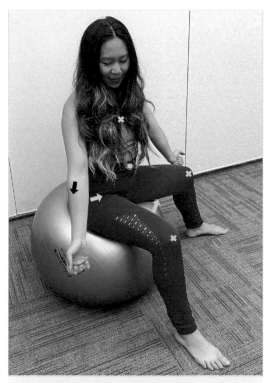

Fig. 13.15 Diagonal muscle fibers contract when the ball is pulled from the right sitting bone toward the left knee.

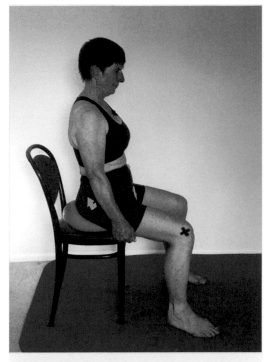

Fig. 13.16 The exercises can be done with a ball "cushion" on a chair.

13.1.6 Bouncing on the Ball

Bouncing increases the pressure exerted on the pelvic floor. Additionally, saying explosive words, such as "kick," "top," and "pow" to name a few, increases intra-abdominal pressure similar to coughing and sneezing (▶ Fig. 13.17). Bouncing may also simulate jumping and running. The goal is to practice coordination of the pelvic floor activity with the activity of the pulmonary diaphragm and the abdominal and back muscles.

- Bounce gently and quickly, contracting the pelvic floor muscles to retrain the fast fibers.
- Breathe in and arch the back. Then exhale, grip the ball, pull it forward, and bounce, lifting off the ball while contracting the pelvic muscles.
- Say explosive words, such as "kick" or "cool," while lifting off the ball.

> **Note**
>
> For safety reasons, exercises are done with the ball in a base, which is a flat dish in which the ball can roll (see ▶ Fig. 12.1), or in a corner, which ensures that the ball does not roll away (▶ Fig. 13.18).

13.1.7 Two People Sitting Back to Back on the Ball

Sitting back to back on the same ball provides the unique possibility to train the pelvic floor muscles eccentrically. One person pulls the ball forward (concentric muscle contraction), while the other person allows the movement to take place but slows it down (eccentric muscle activity). The muscle is strengthened while lengthening, as in how the

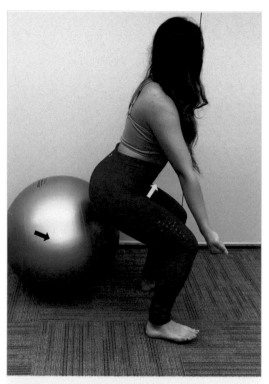

Fig. 13.17 Bouncing on a ball can be done in a corner to ensure that the ball does not roll away. The hands clench when the pelvic floor contracts.

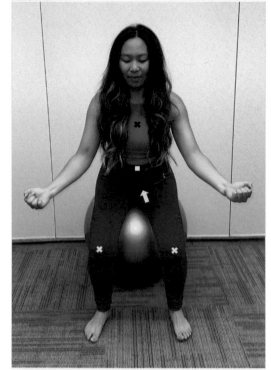

Fig. 13.18 Saying explosive words such as "kick" increases intra-abdominal pressure and, therefore, the challenge.

quadriceps muscle of the leg is strengthened when walking downhill. Starting position is as in ► Fig. 13.19.

The exercises also provide resistance, and pulling against each other improves strength. The competitive aspect can increase the motivation to exercise (► Fig. 13.19).

- One person contracts the pelvic floor muscles during exhalation, moving the ball with the sitting bone in a forward/backward, side to side, or diagonal direction. The other person resists the movement with the pelvic floor muscles (► Fig. 13.19 and ► Fig. 13.20).
- One person moves the ball, and the other person tries to slow down the movement. This movement demands control of the pelvic floor muscles while they lengthen.
- Each partner moves the ball in an opposite direction these are referenced above 13.19 and 13.20.

Note

- The ball has to be big enough to accommodate two people.
- Exercises can be done in different directions of movement.
- Resistive elastic band (TheraBand) is useful for added challenge.
- The exercises can also be done on a double ball.

13.2 Exercises with Resistive Elastic Band (TheraBand)

TheraBand can be used to strengthen the back extensor muscles and the abductor and external rotator muscles of the hips, individually or together, while exercising the pelvic floor muscles (► Fig. 13.20, ► Fig. 13.21, ► Fig. 13.22,

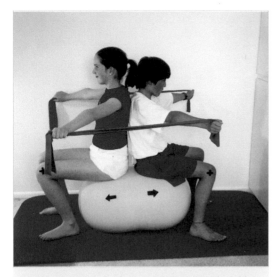

Fig. 13.19 Back to back on a double ball. Both children pull the sitting bones forward while maintaining good posture.

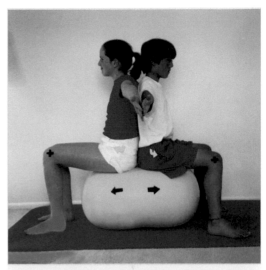

Fig. 13.20 Postural exercises with the upper extremities while exercising the pelvic floor on the double ball.

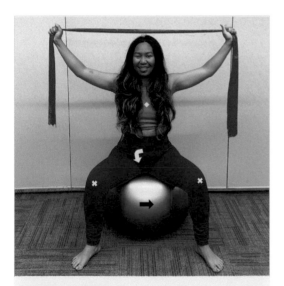

Fig. 13.21 A TheraBand can be used to strengthen the back muscles for preventing osteoporosis.

▶ Fig. 13.23, ▶ Fig. 13.24, ▶ Fig. 13.25, ▶ Fig. 13.26, ▶ Fig. 13.27). The elastic TheraBand comes in various colors and different strengths. It is vital to begin exercising with less resistance at first and then change the resistance to make the exercise more challenging. The yellow band is the most elastic, followed by red, green, blue, black, and silver. Changing to a band that offers

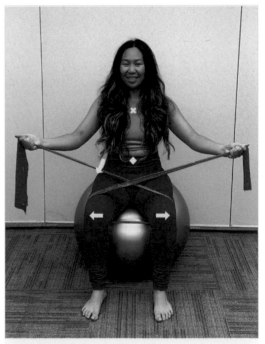

Fig. 13.22 Back extensor and hip abductor muscles are strengthened during the pelvic floor exercises.

more resistance should happen only if the exercise in question is carried out correctly and without substitution.

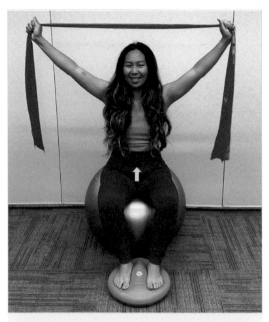

Fig. 13.23 A flat ball under the feet increases the challenge of balancing during the exercise.

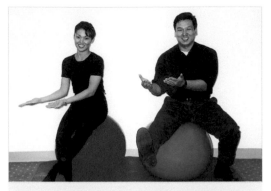

Fig. 13.24 "Cocktail party" exercise. The female shows the starting position, the male the end position.

Including the back extensor muscles in the strengthening program for the pelvic floor assists in improving upright posture and keeping the bones healthy, thus preventing osteoporosis (► Fig. 13.21 and ► Fig. 13.22).

Note

- Increased balance is required if a ball "cushion" is placed under the feet. This progresses the challenge for exercises in a seated position (► Fig. 13.23).
- The "cocktail party" exercise is an adaptation which progresses challenges to balance and strengthens the legs. In ► Fig. 13.24, the woman shows the starting position and the man the end position.[14]
- If adding a TheraBand to this exercise, hold it above the head as in ► Fig. 13.21, while changing the position of the legs from weight-bearing on the right leg to weight-bearing on the left leg. It is essential to first carry out the exercise without the TheraBand and then to increase the challenge. Begin with yellow or red elastic bands and progress to green.

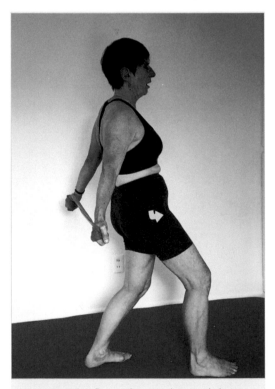

Fig. 13.25 Pelvic floor tightening during exhalation while strengthening the back extensor muscles.

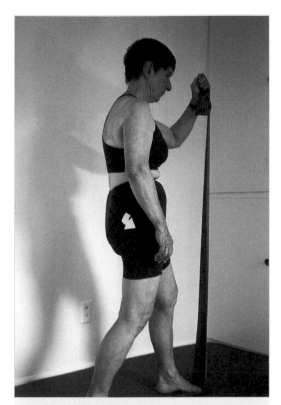

Fig. 13.26 Stepping onto the TheraBand; it is then pulled upward with the arm to strengthen the arm and back muscles.

Refer to ▸ Fig. 13.25, ▸ Fig. 13.26, ▸ Fig. 13.27 for additional exercises using TheraBands.

13.2.1 Exercises in Standing Position

When standing, the pelvic floor is in a horizontal position and has to help carry the load of the viscera. Exercising the pelvic floor can be done with or without a resistive elastic band (TheraBand). A good upright posture with strong pelvic floor muscles is the goal. For osteoporosis prevention, a resistive elastic band can be used to strengthen the back extensor muscles.

- Breathe in while gently arching the back, then breathe out while tightening the pelvic floor muscles.
- Hold the TheraBand behind the back and pull it to the sides during exhalation while tightening the pelvic floor muscles (▸ Fig. 13.25).

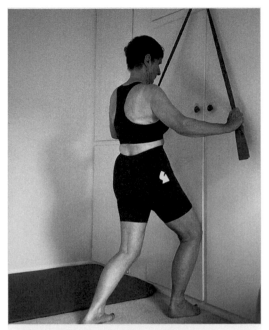

Fig. 13.27 Pulling a TheraBand downward and backward during pelvic floor exercises strengthens the mid back.

- Step onto the TheraBand with one foot and pull it upward and backward while exercising the pelvic floor (▸ Fig. 13.26).
- Hold the TheraBand above the head and pull it to the sides while exercising the pelvic floor.
- Attach the TheraBand to a hook on the wall and pull it downward and backward (▸ Fig. 13.27).
- Stand on a flat ball "cushion," balance board, or trampoline while exercising the pelvic floor muscles (▸ Fig. 13.28).

Note

- Begin in a stepping position with one leg forward.
- Remember that the knees and chest do not move. All the movements come from the pelvis.
- The exercises should be combined with breathing.
- TheraBand can be used to increase the stability of the trunk and to strengthen the back extensors for osteoporosis prevention.

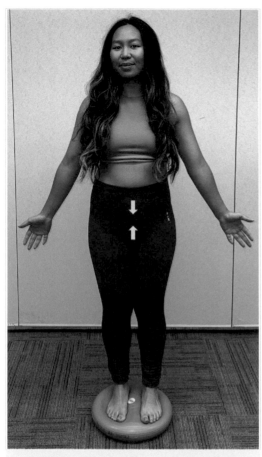

Fig. 13.28 In a standing position, the pelvic floor can be trained while balancing on a ball "cushion." The task is tough with closed eyes.

13.2.2 Challenging Exercises

Many exercises can be adapted to pelvic floor exercises while lying on the back with the knees bent or lying on the stomach. Exercises can also be done while moving from a sitting to a standing position, while rolling from side to side in bed, or when stuck in a traffic jam.

Often favorite exercises can be reviewed and tailored to include the pelvic floor. The following exercises are adaptations of therapeutic exercises by Klein-Vogelbach.[38]

> **Note**
>
> - It is essential to learn to tighten the pelvic floor during functional activities, such as lifting heavy objects, vacuum cleaning, and going upstairs and downstairs, and to coordinate the exercises with breathing.
> - First, learn the task, then coordinate it with breathing, and finally include contraction of the pelvic floor muscles.

The "Frog"

This exercise is challenging and demanding, and easiest to learn in sequences. It functionally trains the abdominal muscles. The rib cage narrows in the end position while the lower abdominal muscles shorten. Breathing coordinates as well.

- In the starting position, inhale and relax the pelvic floor muscles. When moving toward the end position, exhale and contract the pelvic floor.
- First, learn to find the starting position of arms and legs, even with closed eyes (▶ Fig. 13.29). Second, learn the arm movements. Third, practice moving the arms from the starting to the end position (▶ Fig. 13.30).
- Let a therapist correct your posture. The spine should be well aligned. In ▶ Fig. 13.31, the head of the subject is too far forward and not aligned with the trunk.
- The same progression is recommended for the leg movements before the two actions are joined and combined with breathing (also against the resistance of a closed glottis) and pelvic floor contractions (▶ Fig. 13.31).
- In the end position, the heels press together, and the knees move apart (this activates the external rotator muscles of the hips). The pelvis can be lifted off the ground when the heels are pulled in a semicircular movement over the abdomen (▶ Fig. 13.31). The lower

abdominal muscles shorten if the exercise is done correctly.

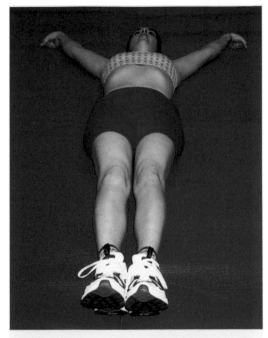

Fig. 13.29 Starting position of the "frog" exercise.

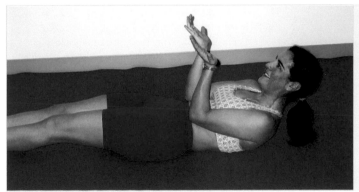

Fig. 13.30 End position of the arm movements of the "frog" exercise.

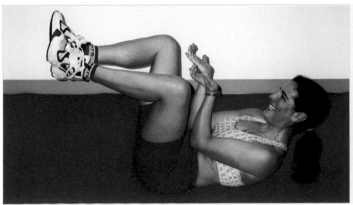

Fig. 13.31 The legs have not yet reached the end position of the "frog." The head is pulled too far forward.

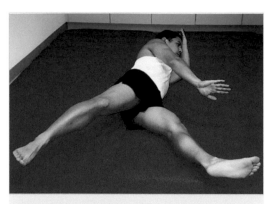

Fig. 13.32 Starting position of the "dreaming police officer." The right heel pushes off the floor.

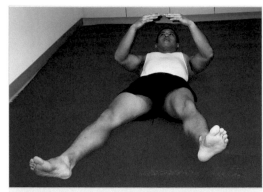

Fig. 13.33 End position of the "dreaming police officer." The feet do not touch the floor.

The "Dreaming Police Officer"

Klein-Vogelbach gave her exercises names that her patients would remember and create a visual image. The following exercise resembles a police officer directing traffic.

During the entire exercise, the spine does not twist or rotate. The rotation takes place in the hip joints. If done correctly, this is a wonderful exercise to improve the stability of the trunk muscles and to strengthen the legs.

- In the starting position, the arms are held in an oval shape in front of the chest (▸ Fig. 13.32). This positioning stabilizes the thorax.
- Spread the legs apart. Push the right heel firmly down onto the floor and turn to the left side, causing the trunk to turn at the hip joints. At the same time, the right arm moves across the body until it is parallel to the left leg. The left arm moves upward next to the head and can be used to stabilize the trunk.
- In the end position, both legs are raised off the ground, with the toes of the front leg pointing upward and those of the back leg pointing downward (▸ Fig. 13.33).

- In the starting position, inhale and relax the pelvic floor muscles; when moving toward the end position, exhale and tighten the pelvic floor muscles.

> **Note**
>
> - In case of difficulty "pushing off" the leg, it may be helpful to place it on a stool or little box.
> - Individuals with a narrow waistline may place a rolled-up towel or small pillow under the waist to increase stability in the end position.
> - If the back is arched too much in the end position, the front leg needs to be moved further forward to increase the "step" size. This action will flatten the lumbar spine.

All the above exercises may be helpful in clients with bladder and bowel dysfunctions. Therapists should always listen attentively to understand which other systems of the body may be involved.

14 Stretching Exercises for the Muscles Surrounding the Pelvic Floor

This chapter demonstrates exercises that can stretch the muscles surrounding the pelvis in a practical way. Thirty-five muscles attach directly to the pelvic girdle and sacrum and contribute to their movement and function.[45] The examples set out here are limited to the muscles listed below because they can influence the position of the pelvis and are significant contributors to pain, imbalances, and poor posture.

- Iliopsoas and rectus femoris muscles
- Hamstring muscles
- Tensor fasciae latae
- Piriformis muscle
- Adductor muscles

Postural alignment of the pelvis in standing, sitting, and kneeling can only be achieved if the muscles are at their proper length. However, scars in the abdominal or hip region, or habits, can cause chronic poor posture (to avoid pain) and this may lead to a shortening of muscles.

As muscle length increases, the opposing muscles or antagonists should strengthen as well (see section The Adductor Muscles [p. 89]).

The ability to maintain a neutral sitting and standing posture is necessary for a well-functioning pelvic floor. Therefore, it is essential to recognize poor posture and associated muscle weakness or shortness and to include gentle mobilization of the scar tissue. A therapist can also determine if there is stiffness (contractures), which cannot be influenced by therapy.

Note

- Poor posture needs to be evaluated because the therapist has to determine which structures can be treated effectively.
- Scars in the abdominal area can cause poor posture and shortening of muscles.
- Being able to achieve a neutral sitting and standing posture effortlessly is essential.
- Lengthening a shortened muscle with daily exercises takes about 6 weeks.
- Stretching should not cause pain (e.g., one should not feel stretch in the low back if the hamstring muscles are stretched).
- Tolerable positions should be selected. Other disabilities, restrictions, or contraindications should be considered.

Example

A woman came for treatment of shoulder and arm pain. The therapist noticed poor postural alignment of the trunk. During the evaluation, the patient stated that she had pelvic floor problems and pain in the lower part of the abdomen. "I have an abdominal scar from a cesarean section and have had pain for 9 years, but my doctor and husband say that I can't have pain because it's only scar tissue. Regardless of what they say, I do have pain, I know it."

Incorporating the abdominal area into the treatment and softening the scar improved not only the client's posture but also eliminated her pain. The hip flexor muscles required stretching as well. They had probably shortened because the client avoided an upright posture (her pectoral muscles of the chest had also shortened).

14.1 Standing and Sitting Correctly for Good Posture

To familiarize yourself with observing posture, examples of suboptimal and improved (not ideal) positions in standing and sitting are demonstrated here. Arrows mark points of observation (► Fig. 14.1, ► Fig. 14.2, ► Fig. 14.3, ► Fig. 14.4).

In ► Fig. 14.1, the arms are placed above the head to allow for better observation of the posture. The lower arrow points to knees that are pushed too far backward; they should be positioned above the midfoot, just in front of the heels, as indicated in ► Fig. 14.2. The pelvis should be in a near-vertical position, as in ► Fig. 14.2. However, the shortness of the iliopsoas muscle and the other hip flexor muscle, the rectus femoris, frequently prevent proper alignment, pulling the pelvis in a forward direction when standing (► Fig. 14.1). Compensation for the forward tilt of the pelvis happens whereby the trunk tends to lean backward. The head is usually positioned over the feet and is therefore pulled forward, as can be observed even in the corrected standing positions.

When sitting, short hamstring muscles tend to tilt the pelvis backward, especially when the knees straighten. The consequence is a flexed lumbar spine and head held in front of the body, the perfect setup for back and neck pain (▶ Fig. 14.3). The corrected sitting posture is shown in ▶ Fig. 14.4. However, this posture can only be maintained for a very short time, unless

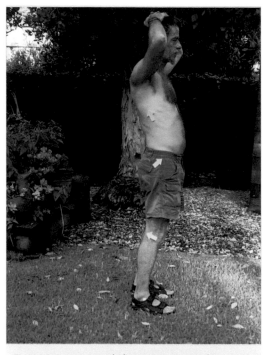

Fig. 14.1 Poor postural alignment in a standing position; arrows indicate the points of observation.

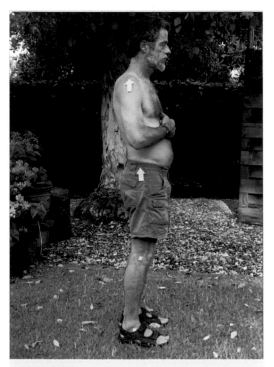

Fig. 14.2 Much improved posture; still not an ideal alignment because of the shortness of the hip flexor muscles.

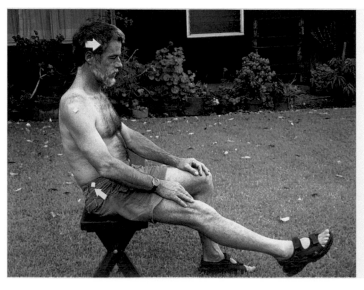

Fig. 14.3 Shortness of hamstring muscles becomes apparent when extending the knee.

all the shortened structures stretch correctly. The tight tensor fasciae latae is visible at the side of the right thigh (▸ Fig. 14.4) and left thigh (▸ Fig. 14.5). The muscle, when tight, also turns the foot outward.

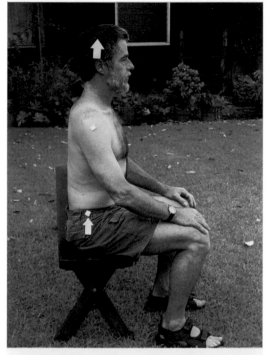

Fig. 14.4 Good sitting posture. However, it does not appear effortless and cannot be maintained because of the shortness of various muscles.

14.2 The Iliopsoas and Rectus Femoris Muscles

- The iliopsoas muscle connects the lumbar spine with the thigh. If short, it can lead to difficulties lying flat on the back. The pelvis is tilted forward, increasing the lumbar lordosis. Pain in the lower abdomen can sometimes be attributed to the iliopsoas muscle. Together with the rectus femoris muscles, it bends (flexes) the hips.
- The rectus femoris muscle is the only part of the quadriceps muscle that connects the pelvis to the lower leg, just below the front of the knee. Therefore, bending the knees while keeping the hips straight when lying flat on the abdomen or kneeling either increases lordosis of the spine or flexion of the thigh in the hip joint. When lying on the back with the feet hanging over the edge of a bench, the knees straighten (extends) to accommodate for the shortness of the muscle. Its shortness can cause pain in the groin and low back because it prevents good posture.

14.2.1 Signs of Shortness of the Hip Flexor Muscles

As shown in ▸ Fig. 14.5 and ▸ Fig. 14.6, the client lies on a bench with the feet hanging over the edge. Shortness of the hip flexor muscles can be recognized by observing the legs. If the thigh is not parallel to the floor, but instead lifted, the iliopsoas muscle is short. If the knee does not

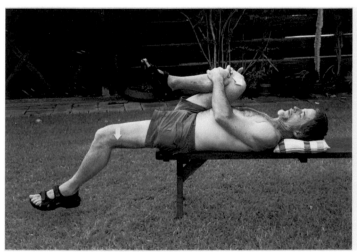

Fig. 14.5 Iliopsoas, rectus femoris, and tensor muscles are tight.

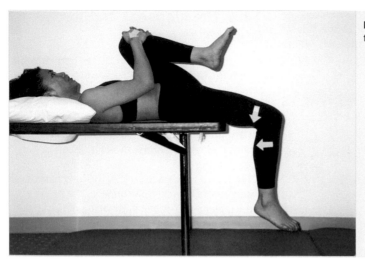

Fig. 14.6 The iliopsoas muscle and the rectus femoris muscle are flexible.

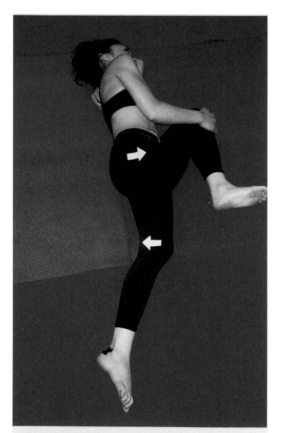

Fig. 14.7 Stretching the right iliopsoas muscle in a side-lying position.

bend at least 90 degrees without lifting the thigh, the rectus femoris muscle is short (▶ Fig. 14.5).

In ▶ Fig. 14.5, the position of the thigh would change if the heel was pulled backward, causing the knee to bend more. The foot of the lower leg is turned outward slightly, probably due to the tightness of the tensor fasciae latae. In ▶ Fig. 14.6, the muscles are flexible, and a neutral standing position can, therefore, be achieved without difficulty.

Moving in the direction of the arrows (▶ Fig. 14.6) can stretch the iliopsoas and rectus femoris muscles. It is important to first bring one knee to the chest to flatten the lumbar spine. To stretch the iliopsoas muscle, the knee can be straight because the muscle does not influence it; it attaches at the thigh close to the hip joint.

14.2.2 Stretching of the Iliopsoas Muscle

- In ▶ Fig. 14.7, the left knee is pulled toward the chest, and the right leg extended backward. The groin moves in a forward direction, and this is where the stretch is felt.
- The stretch (▶ Fig. 14.8) is easy. First, pull one knee to the chest, then try to touch the floor with the thigh of the other leg by pushing the knee downward, extending the leg.
- Lie on the bent knee, face down. The buttock must not move away from the heel while the other leg lifts off the floor (▶ Fig. 14.9).

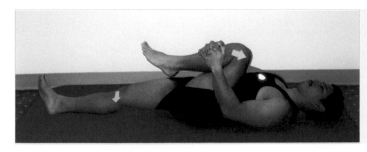

Fig. 14.8 Stretching of the right iliopsoas muscle while lying on the back. Arrows indicate the direction of pull.

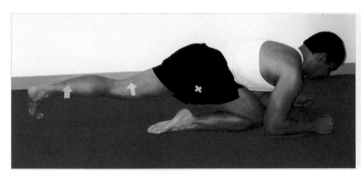

Fig. 14.9 The right buttock should maintain contact with the right heel when trying to lift the left leg. This stretch is difficult; it requires strong hip extensor muscles.

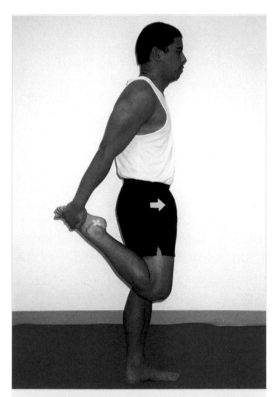

Fig. 14.10 Stretching the rectus femoris muscle while standing. The abdomen stays short, the lumbar spine flat, and the buttock moves away from the heel.

This stretch is difficult, as it demands a flexible iliopsoas and a strong buttock (gluteal) muscle—strong enough to lift the weight of the leg against the tightness of the iliopsoas.

14.2.3 Stretching of the Rectus Femoris Muscle

Functional stretching of the rectus femoris muscle is frequently done incorrectly, stretching the low back rather than the hip.

- When stretching the muscle in standing, it is important to move the buttock away from the heel (▶ Fig. 14.10) and not, as many people do, the heel toward the buttock. The arrows indicate the direction of movement (▶ Fig. 14.10, ▶ Fig. 14.11, ▶ Fig. 14.12, ▶ Fig. 14.13).
- When sitting, it is essential to maintain a backward tilt of the pelvis when moving the knee backward (▶ Fig. 14.11). The abdomen should shorten rather than lengthen between the symphysis pubis and the sternal notch; this helps to keep the lumbar spine flat (▶ Fig. 14.10, ▶ Fig. 14.11, ▶ Fig. 14.12, ▶ Fig. 14.13).

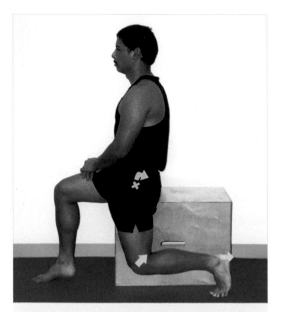

Fig. 14.11 When sitting, the pelvis tilts backward before the knee moves backward.

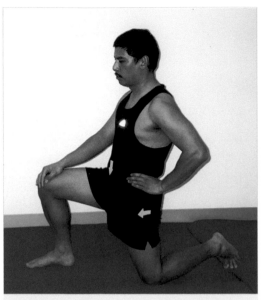

Fig. 14.12 Stretching the rectus muscle in a half-kneeling position. The pelvis is tilted backward, and then the groin moved in a forward direction.

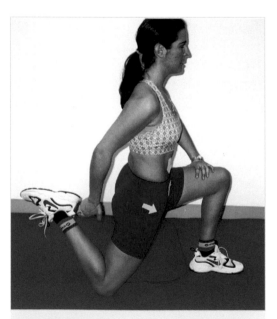

Fig. 14.13 Progression of the rectus femoris stretch (see ▶ Fig. 14.12). The buttock is moved away from the right heel.

14.3 The Hamstring Muscles

The hamstring muscles connect the pelvis to the lower leg, just below the back of the knee. When not at its proper length, the pelvis is tilted backward while sitting, especially when the knee is extended (▶ Fig. 14.3). Therefore, sitting upright on the floor is impossible, unless the knees are bent (▶ Fig. 14.14). The shortness contributes to back and pelvic pain. If one side is tighter than the other, it can cause imbalances.

14.3.1 Signs of Shortness of the Hamstring Muscles

In ▶ Fig. 14.3 and ▶ Fig. 14.14, the shortness of the hamstring muscles is apparent. In ▶ Fig. 14.15, the leg is straightened with ease; the angle at the hip joint between the pelvis and the thigh is approximately 80 degrees, and the leg could be lifted higher without posterior tilting of the pelvis.

When lying on the back, there is shortness of the hamstring muscles if the knee cannot be extended while the thigh is in a near-vertical position of 80 to 90 degrees hip flexion (▶ Fig. 14.16).

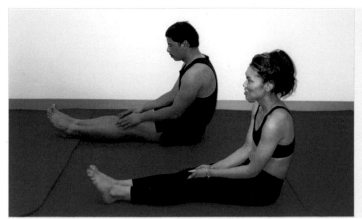

Fig. 14.14 Shortness of the hamstrings prevents sitting upright on the floor.

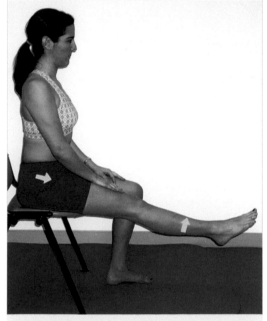

Fig. 14.15 This person sits upright with ease; the hamstring muscles are flexible, and the tensor muscle is not visible at the side.

14.3.2 Stretching of the Hamstring Muscles

- While sitting, tilt the pelvis forward, then lift the lower leg (pull in the direction of the arrows; ▶ Fig. 14.15). The stretching "pain" can be felt behind the knee. The back should never hurt.
- It is essential to prestretch the proximal end of the hamstring muscles near the hips (▶ Fig. 14.17 and ▶ Fig. 14.18).

The stretch should be gentle and in the direction of the arrow.
- First, move the pelvis in a forward direction, then straighten the knee (▶ Fig. 14.18 and ▶ Fig. 14.19). Feel the stretch behind the knee.

14.4 The Tensor Fasciae Latae Muscle

The tensor fasciae latae muscle originates at the pelvis, near the rectus femoris muscle, and attaches at the side of the lower leg, just below the knee. To accommodate for its shortness, a person tends to sit with the legs apart, sometimes with the feet turned outward. The muscle, which has a small muscle belly and a large fascia, can contribute to imbalances of the pelvic girdle and pain. The pain is reported near the groin and described as pressure and tightness at the side of the hips (below the "x" in ▶ Fig. 14.21).

14.4.1 Signs of Shortness of the Tensor Fasciae Latae

When hanging over the edge of a bench (not a position for everybody with a short tensor muscle), shortness of the tensor fasciae latae becomes apparent through the position of the leg in the air. Trying to pull it toward the ground already stretches the muscle (▶ Fig. 14.20). In ▶ Fig. 14.21, the muscle is less tight than in the previous figure. The man in ▶ Fig. 14.20 sits with the legs apart because the tensor muscle is so tight. This tightness can cause pain, usually presenting as pressure below the area marked with an "x" in ▶ Fig. 14.21 or as pain in the groin area.

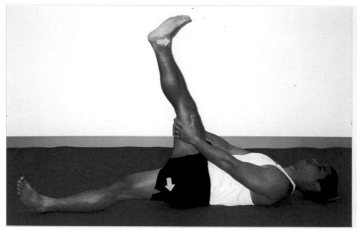

Fig. 14.16 When straightening the leg to stretch the hamstrings, the thigh should be in a near-vertical position. The opposite knee should not lift off the floor.

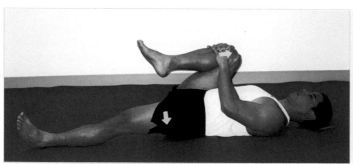

Fig. 14.17 Prestretch of the hamstring muscle; the knee is pulled toward the chest while the other knee is kept down, which will automatically stretch the iliopsoas muscle on the opposite side.

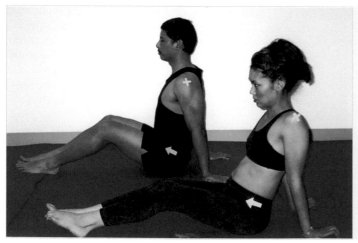

Fig. 14.18 First, the pelvis is moved forward while the knees are bent.

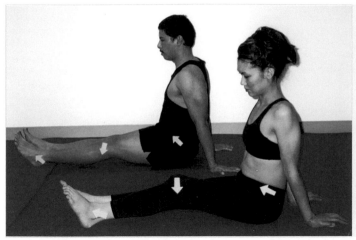

Fig. 14.19 The knees are slowly straightened while keeping the pelvis tilted forward (see arrows).

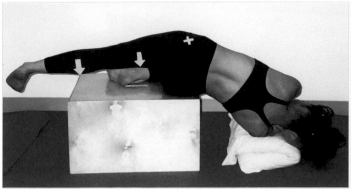

Fig. 14.20 The tight tensor fasciae latae keeps the left leg high in the air.

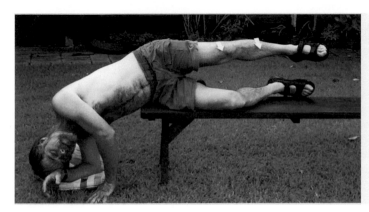

Fig. 14.21 In this person, the tensor muscle is longer and is closer to the ground.

14.4.2 Stretching of the Tensor Fasciae

There are various ways of stretching the tensor muscle. The stretch illustrated here was selected because it demonstrates the tightness well (▶ Fig. 14.20 and ▶ Fig. 14.21). Moreover, the muscle can stretch itself in this way, provided that the head-down position (trunk hanging over the side of the bench) is tolerable. Because the weight

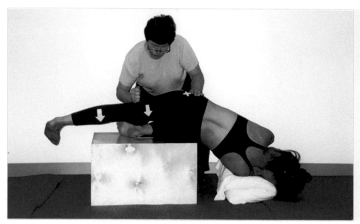

Fig. 14.22 The tensor fasciae latae is stretched by a therapist by applying pressure with the hand.

of the trunk stabilizes the pelvis, performing the movement incorrectly, whether voluntarily or involuntarily, is less natural. Often one or two treatments can reduce the nagging pain which the shortness of the tensor fasciae latae can cause.

If this position is not tolerable, the muscle can be stretched in standing:

- Cross the right foot in front of the left one, then lean the trunk to the left with the arm elevated. However, it is easy to perform the movement incorrectly, whether subconsciously or consciously, to avoid pain or strain.
- In side-lying position, the adductor muscles of the same leg can be engaged by actively pulling the leg toward the ground (▶ Fig. 14.21; arrows show the direction of pull).
- In side-lying position, a therapist can apply gentle pressure and use the hand to gently stretch the side of the leg (▶ Fig. 14.22).
- The tensor stretch can be combined with the stretch of the iliopsoas and rectus femoris muscle if the knee is pulled toward the middle (see ▶ Fig. 14.5 and ▶ Fig. 14.6 as well as ▶ Fig. 14.23).

14.5 The Piriformis Muscle

The piriformis muscle originates at the sacrum and attaches to the thigh. The muscle helps to stabilize the sacroiliac joints and tends to imitate sciatic pain when tight. The pain is usually felt at the center of the buttock or may be referred to the lower part of the back where the sacrum and the ileum join. Stretching this muscle can also mobilize the sacroiliac joint.

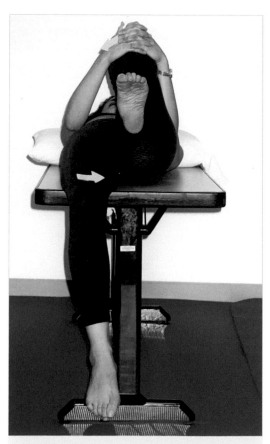

Fig. 14.23 Lying on the back with the lower leg hanging over the edge of the bench, the tensor fasciae latae is stretched if the bent knee is pulled toward the middle.

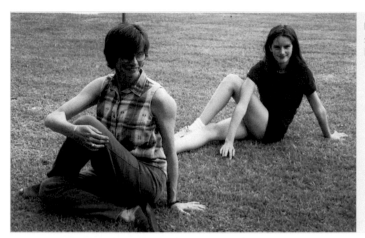

Fig. 14.24 Demonstration of a well-stretched piriformis muscle of the left buttock.

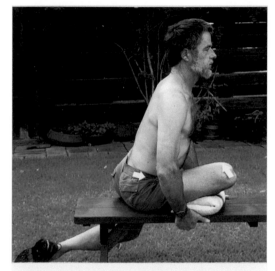

Fig. 14.25 Stretching the piriformis; the trunk is leaning over the leg.

14.5.2 Stretching of the Piriformis

- The thigh can be pulled toward the chest with the hand or the elbow of the opposite arm (▶ Fig. 14.24). The stretch increases if the posture is correct, that is, when the trunk is erect. The buttock muscle (gluteal muscles) and certain parts of the abductor muscles, which generally pull the legs to the sides, are also stretched.
- Try positioning the leg on a pillow and stretching the piriformis muscle by leaning the trunk forward (▶ Fig. 14.25 and ▶ Fig. 14.26). Since most of these stretches also mobilize the sacroiliac joints, it is important to be cautious with people who have complaints in this area and ensure that exercises are done gently and carefully.

14.6 The Adductor Muscles

The adductor muscles consist of a group of short and long muscles. It is important to remember that their attachment is at the pelvis. It is at the center and the front of the seat. Therefore, this muscle group can pull the symphysis pubis upward or downward on one side, causing pain in the center of the seat. Equally, tightening of the adductor muscles on one side may also correct an asymmetry at the symphysis pubis. The muscles form the inside of the thigh, and portions attach below the knee, on the inside of the leg. Spreading of the legs, therefore, stretches the adductor muscles. It is normal

14.5.1 Signs of Tightness of the Piriformis Muscle

Observing how easily the left leg can be pulled toward the erect trunk (▶ Fig. 14.24) shows what kind of movement is achievable with a well-stretched piriformis. If this is difficult to do or the left buttock lifts, the piriformis is probably short. Stretching pain can be felt across the buttock.

to be able to move the leg approximately 50 degrees to the side (▶ Fig. 14.27).

14.6.1 Stretching of the Adductor Muscles

- Sit on the floor with the legs spread apart. Keep the legs apart as you lean forward, or lean toward one leg or the other.

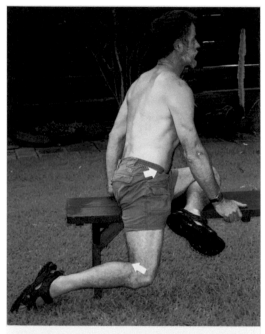

Fig. 14.26 The piriformis muscle stretch also mobilizes the sacroiliac joint.

- Lying on the back, bend the knees, then lower the thighs in the direction of the floor. The feet touch with the soles.
- There are many different ways of stretching the adductor muscles. The ultimate stretch is, of course, the splits, even though this should not be the goal for the average person.
- Of course, actively pulling the legs apart helps to stretch the adductor muscles, which are inhibited by the action of the antagonist. (▶ Video 14.1, ▶ Video 14.2, ▶ Video 14.3, ▶ Video 14.4, and ▶ Video 14.5)

To stretch the hip flexor muscles, the hip extensor muscles need to be strengthened (see ▶ Fig. 14.9 and ▶ Fig. 14.10). The quadriceps need to be strengthened to stretch the hamstring muscles

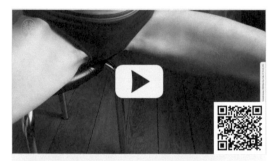

Video 14.1 Example of abnormal adductor tone

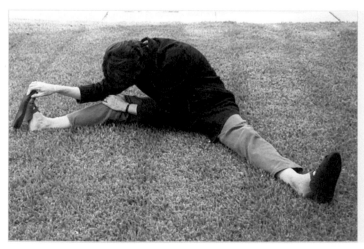

Fig. 14.27 Stretching the adductor muscles.

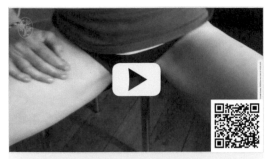

Video 14.2 Corrective adductor stretch of side

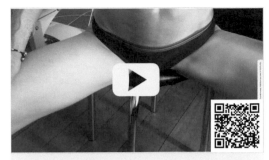

Video 14.3 Corrective adductor stretch with forward lean

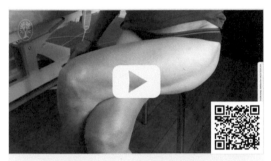

Video 14.4 Adductor mobilization of left

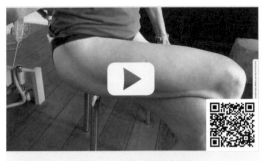

Video 14.5 Adductor mobilization of right

(see ► Fig. 14.15). The hip adductor muscles need to be strengthened to improve the tensor fasciae latae and the length of the hip abductor muscles (see ► Fig. 14.20 and ► Fig. 14.21). If the external rotator muscles of the hips are short and weak, internal rotation of the hips has to be strengthened by actively pulling the leg toward the trunk (see ► Fig. 14.24). The hip abductor muscles improve adductor length by actively pulling the legs gently apart.

For them to be effective, stretches must be performed precisely. Opinions on how long to stretch differs and can vary depending on what muscle types the stretches are targeting. However, most important is that the stretching is combined with an awareness training about good and bad posture. If the stretching is combined with frequent attempts to optimize posture, there will be a much better chance for permanent improvement.

Appendix A

Physical Therapy Evaluation of Female Incontinence

Name:
Date:
Date of birth:
Health insurance:
MD:
Therapist:
Diagnosis:
Previous therapy? Yes/No. When?_____

Surgical history (please circle if applicable):

- Abdominal surgeries _____
- Hernia. Location? _____
- Appendix
- Gallbladder
- Laparoscopy
- Hemorrhoids
- Other _____

Childbirth information

- Number of pregnancies?
- Number of births?
- Weight of heaviest child?
- How many hours was the longest labor?
- Cesarean section?
- Episiotomy?
- Natural tearing?
- Bladder suspension surgery?
- Hysterectomy?
- Other? _____

Medical history

- Diabetes   yes/no
- Heart problems   yes/no
- Cancer   yes/no
- Bladder infections   yes/no
- History of bed-wetting   yes/no
- Other _____

Medication

- Are you currently taking any form of medication? _____

Current symptoms

What new or ongoing symptoms are you experiencing?

- Urinary frequency
- Sudden or strong urge to urinate: AM/PM/BOTH
- Incomplete emptying
- Accidental leakage (please circle if applicable):
  - Exercising
  - Coughing
  - Sneezing
  - Straining
  - Running
  - Going upstairs or downstairs
  - Resting
  - During intercourse
  - Performing any other activities (e.g., standing up, turning, jumping, weight lifting)

Do you experience (please circle if applicable):

- Bladder or pelvic pain
- Hesitancy
- Urgencies
- Need to push/strain when urinating
- Stool leakage
- Constipation
- Sexual dysfunction

How often do you have to urinate?

- During the day:
- At night:

Do you have any pain?
(e.g., during urination or intercourse)
If yes, please describe: _____

How long have you had these symptoms?_____

Have you had success with any interventions reducing your symptoms?_____

On a scale of 1–10 (10 being the most, 1 the least), how much do your symptoms impact your daily life? Circle one:

1   2   3   4   5   6   7   8   9   10

Do you use one of the following during the day or at night?
(Please circle if applicable and indicate amount)

- Liners   day/night _____
- Pads   day/night _____
- Adult protection   day/night _____

Daily fluid intake:_____ glasses/mL
How many cups or glasses of the following do you drink daily?

- Water   _____
- Alcohol   _____
- Coffee   _____
- Citrus juice   _____
- Tea   _____
- Fruit juice   _____
- Soda   _____
- Other   _____

Bowel habits

- Regular (1–3/day)   yes/no
- Bowel incontinence   yes/no
- Gas   yes/no
- Constipation   yes/no
- Diarrhea   yes/no
- Do you use laxatives?   yes/no
- Do you have a fiber-rich diet?   yes/no

History of treatment

- Have you previously been treated for this condition?   yes/no
- Have you previously done Kegel or any other pelvic exercises?   yes/no
- Other treatments?   yes/no
- Which ones? _____
- If they were effective, how did your symptoms change?
_____

Psychosocial history

• Current/previous employment? Lifting involved with job or home life?
_____

• Hobbies:
• Sports:

How do you define health?_____

What is your treatment goal?_____

To be completed by the therapist

Objective Findings:

• Posture
  - Pelvic alignment
  - Muscle imbalances around pelvic girdle
• Breathing patterns
  - Coordination of pelvic and thoracic dia-
phragms
  - Ability to perform diaphragmatic breathing
• Abdomen
  - Scars, fascial patterns, lines of tension or tightness, soft tissue tone
  - Active Straight Leg Raise (Strength/Stability)
• Pelvic mobility and coordination with transversus abdominus
• Ability to "feel" the activity of pelvic floor muscles
• Able to contract without overuse of the gluteal muscles

Pelvic Floor Assessment:

• Visual screen of external perineum:
  - Perineal body above or below horizontal line between ischial tuberosities
  - Introitus gap?
  - Anterior or posterior bulge?
  - Urethral position. Retracted? Descended? Protruding?
  - Skin color, texture, health
• Visual assessment of pelvic floor muscles externally:
  - Observation of contraction/relaxation, note timing, recruitment and control.
  - Cough reflex?
  - Pelvic clock palpation—note tone differences at clock positions
  - Cotton swab test

Intravaginal Muscle/Soft Tissue Assessment:

• Muscle tone at superficial triangle first then deeper
• Strength of pelvic floor and surrounding muscles at superficial and deeper positions
  - Obturator internus, ischiococcygeus, iliococcygeus, and puburectalis
  - Phasic ability (contract/relax 10 times as fast as possible—"quick flicks")
  - Tonic ability (hold contraction for 10 seconds) number of seconds held/intensity decline
  - Co-contraction of transversus abdominus, impact?
  - Overflow into adductors or gluteals?
• Prolapse with bearing down. Grade 1–4.

Impairment(s):

• Poor sensory awareness of pelvic floor muscles
• Dyscoordination of breathing
• Tightness of iliopsoas muscles

Functional Limitation(s):

• Inability to extend the hips
• Poor posture
• Loss of urine when getting out of the car

Disability/Activities of Daily Living (ADL) Limitation:

• Inability to hold urine for more than 1 hour
• Inability to participate in sports, go to a movie, or go shopping

Goal(s):

• Seeing a movie without losing urine
• Holding urine for 2 hours when shopping

Plan/Intervention:

• Breathing exercises
• Sensory awareness training
• Stretching exercises
• Strengthening exercises for the pelvic floor and surrounding muscles

Date/Signature:

Appendix B

Physical Therapy Evaluation of Male Incontinence

Name:
Date of birth:
Diagnosis:
Date therapy begun:
Health insurance:
MD:
Therapist:

Surgical history (please circle if applicable):

- Abdominal surgeries
- Hernia
- Appendix
- Gallbladder
- Laparoscopy
- Hemorrhoids
- Prostatectomy
- Other

Medical history

- Diabetes   yes/no
- Heart problems   yes/no
- Cancer   yes/no
- Bladder infections   yes/no
- History of bed-wetting   yes/no
- Other _____

What new or ongoing symptoms are you experiencing?

- Urinary frequency
- Sudden or strong urge to urinate: AM/PM/BOTH
- Incomplete emptying
- Dribbling urine?
- Erectile dysfunction?
- Difficulty urinating because of stricture (scar tissue in the urethra)? (If so, is your doctor aware of the problem? Were any procedures undertaken?)

Accidental leakage
(please circle if applicable):

- Exercising
- Coughing
- Sneezing
- Straining
- Performing any other activities (e.g., standing up, turning, jumping, weight lifting)
- Running
- Going upstairs or downstairs
- Resting
- During intercourse

Do you experience
(please circle if applicable):

- Bladder or pelvic pain
- Hesitancy
- Urgencies
- Need to push/strain when urinating
- Stool leakage
- Constipation
- Sexual dysfunction

When urinating do you sit or stand? Please circle.

How often do you have to urinate?

- During the day?
- At night?

Do you have any pain? (during urination or intercourse)

If yes, please describe:_____

How long have you had these symptoms?

Have you had success with any interventions reducing your symptoms?

On a scale of 1–10 (10 being the most, 1 the least), how much do your symptoms impact your daily life? Circle one:

1   2   3   4   5   6   7   8   9   10

Do you use one of the following during the day or at night?
(Please circle if applicable and indicate amount.)

- Liners   day/night _____
- Pads   day/night _____
- Adult protection   day/night _____

Daily fluid intake: glasses/mL

How many cups or glasses of the following do you drink daily?

- Water   _____
- Alcohol   _____
- Coffee   _____
- Citrus juice   _____
- Tea   _____
- Fruit juice   _____
- Soda   _____
- Other   _____

Bowel habits

- Regular (1–3/day)   yes/no
- Bowel incontinence   yes/no
- Gas   yes/no
- Constipation   yes/no
- Diarrhea   yes/no
- Do you use laxatives?   yes/no
- Do you have a fiber-rich diet?   yes/no

History of treatment

- Have you previously been treated for this condition?   yes/no
- Have you previously done Kegel or any other pelvic exercises?   yes/no
- Other treatments?   yes/no
- Which ones?_____
- If they were effective, how did your symptoms change?_____

Psychosocial history

- Current/previous employment? Lifting involved with job or home life?
- Hobbies:
- Sports:

How do you define health?_____

What is your treatment goal?_____

To be filled out by the therapist

Objective Findings:

- Posture
  - Pelvic alignment
  - Muscle imbalances around pelvic girdle
- Breathing patterns
  - Coordination of pelvic and thoracic diaphragms
  - Ability to perform diaphragmatic breathing
- Abdomen
  - Scars, fascial patterns, lines of tension or tightness, soft tissue tone
  - Active Straight Leg Raise (Strength/Stability)
- Pelvic mobility and coordination with transversus abdominus
- Ability to "feel" the activity of pelvic floor muscles
  - Able to contract without overuse of the gluteal muscles

Impairment(s):

- Poor sensory awareness of pelvic floor muscles
- Dyscoordination of breathing
- Tightness of iliopsoas muscles

Functional Limitation(s):

- Inability to extend the hips
- Poor posture
- Loss of urine when getting out of the car

Disability/ADL Limitation:

- Inability to hold urine for more than 1 hour
- Inability to participate in sports, go to a movie, or go shopping

Goal(s):

- Seeing a movie without losing urine
- Holding urine for 2 hours when shopping

Plan/Intervention:

- Breathing exercises
- Sensory awareness training
- Stretching exercises
- Strengthening exercises for the pelvic floor and surrounding muscles

Date/Signature:

Appendix C

Physical Therapy Evaluation of Male Patients Scheduled for or Post Prostate Surgery

Name:
Date:
Date of birth:
Diagnosis:
Date of diagnosis:
Date of surgery:
Type of surgery:
Health insurance:
MD:
Therapist:

Surgical history
(please circle if applicable):
- Abdominal surgeries
- Hernia
- Appendix
- Gallbladder
- Laparoscopy
- Hemorrhoids
- Other

Medical history

- Diabetes   yes/no
- Heart problem   yes/no
- Cancer   yes/no
- Radiation   yes/no
- Chemotherapy   yes/no
- Bladder infections   yes/no
- History of bed-wetting   yes/no
- Other

Medication

- Are you currently taking any form of medication?

What new or ongoing symptoms are you experiencing?

- **Urinary frequency**
- **Sudden or strong urge to urinate:** AM/PM/**BOTH Incomplete emptying**

- Dribbling urine
- Erectile dysfunction

- Difficulty urinating because of stricture (scar tissue in the urethra)? (If so, is your doctor aware of the problem? Were any procedures undertaken?)

Accidental leakage
(please circle if applicable):

- Exercising
- Coughing
- Sneezing
- Straining
- Performing any other activities (e.g., standing up, turning, jumping, weight lifting)?
- Running
- Going upstairs or downstairs
- Resting
- During intercourse

Do you experience
(please circle if applicable):

- Bladder or pelvic pain
- Hesitancy
- Urgencies
- Need to push/strain when urinating
- Stool leakage
- Constipation
- Sexual dysfunction

When urinating do you sit or stand? Please circle.

How often do you have to urinate?
- During the day?
- At night?

Do you have any pain? (during urination or intercourse)

If yes, please describe:_____

How long have you had these symptoms?

Have you had success with any interventions reducing your symptoms?

On a scale of 1–10 (10 being the most, 1 the least), how much do your symptoms impact your daily life? Circle one:

1   2   3   4   5   6   7   8   9   10

Do you use one of the following during the day or at night?
(Please circle if applicable and indicate amount)

- Liners   day/night _____
- Pads   day/night _____
- Adult protection   day/night _____

Daily fluid intake: glasses/mL

How many cups or glasses of the following do you drink daily?

- Water   _____
- Alcohol   _____
- Coffee   _____
- Citrus juice   _____
- Tea   _____
- Fruit juice   _____
- Soda   _____
- Other   _____

Bowel habits

- Regular (1–3/day)   yes/no
- Bowel incontinence   yes/no
- Gas   yes/no
- Constipation   yes/no
- Diarrhea   yes/no
- Do you use laxatives?   yes/no
- Do you have a fiber-rich diet?   yes/no

History of treatment

- Have you previously been treated for this condition?   yes/no
- Have you previously done Kegel or any other pelvic exercises?   yes/no
- Other treatments?   yes/no
- Which ones?_____
- If they were effective, how did your symptoms change?

Psychosocial history

- Current/previous employment? Lifting involved with job or home life?
- Hobbies:
- Sports:

How do you define health?_____

What is your treatment goal?_____

Plan/intervention:

One or two individual or group treatments before surgery. Reevaluation when the catheter is removed.

Date/signature of physical therapist:

Appendix D

Reevaluation Post Prostate Surgery

Name:
Date:
Date of birth:
Health insurance:
MD:
Therapist:
Diagnosis:
Date catheter removed:

- Were there any surgical complications?   yes/no
- Is follow-up radiation or chemotherapy scheduled?   yes/no

- If taking medications at present, please list:

- Any change in medical status?   yes/no
- Do you have pain?   yes/no

- How much and what do you drink? (Note that coffee, tea, juice of citrus fruits, alcohol, and soda can cause frequent urination.)
- Do you have any difficulty urinating because of strictures (scar tissue in urinary tract)?   yes/no

What new or ongoing symptoms are you experiencing?

- Urinary frequency
- Sudden or strong urge to urinate: AM/PM/BOTH
- Incomplete emptying
- Dribbling urine?
- Erectile dysfunction?
- Difficulty urinating because of stricture (scar tissue in the urethra)? (If so, is your doctor aware of the problem? Were any procedures undertaken?)

Accidental leakage (please circle if applicable):

- Exercising
- Coughing
- Sneezing
- Straining
- Performing any other activities (e.g., standing up, turning, jumping, weight lifting)
- Running
- Going upstairs or downstairs
- Resting
- During intercourse

Do you experience (please circle if applicable):

- Bladder or pelvic pain
- Hesitancy
- Urgencies
- Need to push/strain when urinating
- Stool leakage
- Constipation
- Sexual dysfunction

When urinating do you sit or stand? Please circle.

How often do you have to urinate?

- During the day?
- At night?

Do you have any pain?
(during urination or intercourse)

If yes, please describe:_____

How long have you had these symptoms?

Have you had success with any interventions reducing your symptoms?

On a scale of 1–10 (10 being the most, 1 the least), how much do your symptoms impact your daily life? Circle one:

| 1 | 2 | 3 | 4 | 5 | 6 | 7 | 8 | 9 | 10 |

Do you use one of the following during the day or at night? (Please circle if applicable and indicate amount)

- Liners   day/night _____
- Pads   day/night _____
- Adult protection day/night _____

Daily fluid intake: glasses/mL

How many cups or glasses of the following do you drink daily?

- Water   _____
- Alcohol   _____
- Coffee   _____
- Citrus juice _____
- Tea   _____
- Fruit juice _____
- Soda   _____
- Other   _____

Bowel habits

- Regular (1–3/day)   yes/no
- Bowel incontinence   yes/no
- Gas   yes/no
- Constipation   yes/no
- Diarrhea   yes/no
- Do you use laxatives?   yes/no
- Do you have a fiber-rich diet? yes/no

History of treatment

- Have you previously been treated for this condition?   yes/no
- Have you previously done Kegel or any other pelvic exercises?   yes/no
- Other treatments?   yes/no
- Which ones?_____
- If they were effective, how did your symptoms change?
_____

Psychosocial history

- Current/previous employment? Lifting involved with job or home life?
- Hobbies:
- Sports:

How do you define health?_____

What is your goal for treatment?_____

When did you resume exercising after the surgery?

- Do you have a sensory awareness of:

- – Your pelvic floor   yes/no
- – Your sphincter muscles   yes/no
- Do you exercise?   yes/no

- How often do you exercise? Daily?
- Do the exercises help?   yes/no

- Do you perform breathing exercises in combination with the pelvic floor exercises?

How often do you exercise? _____Daily? _____

Date/Signature: _____

Appendix E

Voiding Diary

Time	Urine in toilet	Urine leakage with activity (cough, laugh, jump)	Urine leakage with urge to empty bladder	Urge to empty bladder without leakage	Fluid intake: amount and type
12 am–1 am					
1 am–2 am					
2					
3					
4					
5					
6					
7					
8					
9					
10					
11					
12					
1 pm					
2					
3					
4					
5					
6					
7					
8					
9					
10					
11					
12					

Indicate events with an "X" in the box.

Suggested Reading

[1] American Physical Therapy Association. Guide to Physical Therapist Practice. Part 1: A description of patient/client management. Part 2: Preferred practice patterns. Phys Ther. 1997; 77(11):1160–1656

[2] Baessler K, Bell BE. Alternative methods to pelvic floor muscle awareness and training. In: Baessler K, Burgio KL, Norton PA, Schüssler B, Moore KH, Stanton SL, eds. Pelvic Floor Re-education. London: Springer; 2008:208–212

[3] Baumann M, Tauber B. Inkontinenz beim Mann. Krankengymnastik. 1991; 12(43):1372–1386

[4] Bo K, Berghmans B, Morkved S, van Kampen M. Evidence-Based Physical Therapy for the Pelvic Floor. Elsevier; 2007

[5] Bø K, Kvarstein B, Nygaard I. Lower urinary tract symptoms and pelvic floor muscle exercise adherence after 15 years. Obstet Gynecol. 2005; 105(5 Pt 1):999–1005

[6] Calais-Germain B. The Female Pelvis Anatomy & Exercises. Eastland Press; 2003

[7] Cantieni B. Tiger Feeling. Suedwest Verlag; 2003

[8] Cantieni B. Tiger feeling. Das sinnliche Beckenbodentraining. 7th ed. Berlin: Verlag Gesundheit; 1998

[9] Cantieni B. Tigerfeeling: The Perfect Pelvic Floor Training for Men and Women. Südwest Verlag; 2013

[10] Cantieni B. Tiger Feeling. The Sensual Pelvic Floor Training for Her and Him. 2000

[11] Carrière B. Functional exercises for the pelvic floor. Video. Denver: Ball dynamics; 1999. www.balldynamics.com

[12] Carrière B. Strengthening the pelvic floor muscles. Physical Therapy Products. 1999; 9:48–50

[13] Carrière B. The Pelvic Floor. Thieme; 2006

[14] Carrière B. The Swiss Ball. Berlin-New York: Springer Verlag; 1998

[15] Clemons N, Poe J. Meditations for Pelvic Health. Portland Pelvic Therapy. Audio CD

[16] Donatelli Ihm J, Lavender M. Below Your Belt: How to Be Queen of Your Pelvic Region. Women's Health Foundation; 2015

[17] Dorey G. Conservative Treatment of Male Urinary Incontinence and Erectile Dysfunction. London: Whurr Publishers Ltd.; 2001

[18] Dorey G. Pelvic Dysfunction in Men. John Wiley & Sons, Ltd.; 2006

[19] Elbadawi A. Pathology and pathophysiology of detrusor in incontinence. Urol Clin North Am. 1995; 22(3):499–512

[20] Fantl JA, Newman DK, Colling J, et al. Managing acute and chronic urinary incontinence, clinical practice guideline. No. 2, 1996 update. Rockville MD, US Department of Health and Human Services; 1996

[21] Fantl JA, Newman DK, Colling J, et al. Urinary incontinence in adults: acute and chronic management. Clinical practice guideline, no. 2, 1996 update. Rockville, MD: Agency for Healthcare Policy and Research, Public Health Service, U. p. Department of Health and Human Services; 1996

[22] Feng M, Parekh A, Bremner H, Kirages D, Kaswick J, Aboseif P. The role of pelvic floor exercise on postprostatectomy incontinence. Unpublished study presented at the American Urology Conference, Atlanta; 2000

[23] Franklin E. Pelvic Power: Mind/Body Exercises for Strength, Flexibility, Posture, and Balance for Men and Women. Elysian editions, Princeton Book Company; 2002

[24] Golmakani N, Zare Z, Khadem N, Shareh H, Shakeri MT. The effect of pelvic floor muscle exercises program on sexual self-efficacy in primiparous women after delivery. Iran J Nurs Midwifery Res. 2015; 20(3):347–353

[25] Guide to physical therapist practice. 2nd ed. American Physical Therapy Association. Phys Ther. 2001; 81(1):9–746

[26] Handa VL, Blomquist JL, Knoepp LR, Hoskey KA, McDermott KC, Muñoz A. Pelvic floor disorders 5–10 years after vaginal or cesarean childbirth. Obstet Gynecol. 2011; 118(4):777–784

[27] Handa VL, Cundiff G, Chang HH, Helzlsouer KJ. Female sexual function and pelvic floor disorders. Obstet Gynecol. 2008; 111(5):1045–1052

[28] Handa VL, Harris TA, Ostergard DR. Protecting the pelvic floor: obstetric management to prevent incontinence and pelvic organ prolapse. Obstet Gynecol. 1996; 88(3):470–478

[29] Havig K. The health care experiences of adult survivors of child sexual abuse: a systematic review of evidence on sensitive practice. Trauma Violence Abuse. 2008; 9(1):19–33

[30] Heller A. Geburtsvorbereitung. Stuttgart: Thieme Verlag; 1998

[31] Heller A. Nach der Geburt. Stuttgart: Thieme Verlag in press; 2001

[32] Hüter-Becker A, Thom H. Massage, Kolonbehandlung. Physiotherapie. 1996; 6:162–182

[33] Jette AM. Physical disablement concepts for physical therapy research and practice. Phys Ther. 1994; 74(5): 380–386

[34] Jette AM. Physical disablement concepts for physical therapy research and practice. Phys Ther. 1994; 74(5):380–386

[35] Kegel AH. Progressive resistance exercise in the functional restoration of the perineal muscles. Am J Obstet Gynecol. 1948; 56(2):238–248

[36] Klein-Vogelbach P. Functional Kinetics. Ball Exercises Videotape. Berlin-Heidelberg-New York: Springer Verlag; 1990

[37] Klein-Vogelbach P. Therapeutic Exercises in Functional Kinetics. Berlin-Heidelberg-New York: Springer Verlag; 1991

[38] Klein-Vogelbach (1992)

[39] Klein-Vogelbach (2000)

[40] Komesu YM, Schrader RM, Ketai LH, Rogers RG, Dunivan GC. Epidemiology of mixed, stress, and urgency urinary incontinence in middle-aged/older women: the importance of incontinence history. Int Urogynecol J Pelvic Floor Dysfunct. 2016; 27(5):763–772

[41] Lara LA, Montenegro ML, Franco MM, Abreu DC, Rosa e Silva AC, Ferreira CH. Is the sexual satisfaction of postmenopausal women enhanced by physical exercise and pelvic floor muscle training? J Sex Med. 2012; 9(1):218–223

[42] Laycock J, Haslam J. Therapeutic Management of Incontinence and Pain

[43] Laycock J, Jerwood D. Pelvic floor muscle assessment: the perfect scheme. Physiotherapy. 2001; 87:631–642

[44] Lee DG. 1999. The pelvic girdle. 2nd ed. Churchill Livingstone Edinburgh

[45] Lee DG. The Pelvic Girdle: An Integration of Clinical Expertise and Research. 4th ed. Edinburgh: Churchill Livingstone; 2011

[46] Massery M. Multisystem consequences of impaired breathing mechanics and/or postural control. In: Frownfelter D, Dean E, eds. Cardiovascular and Pulmonary Physical Therapy Evidence and Practice. 4th ed. St. Louis, MO: Elsevier Health Sciences; 2006:695–717

[47] Massery M, Hagins M, Stafford R, Moerchen V, Hodges PW. Effect of airway control by glottal structures on postural stability. J Appl Physiol (1985). 2013; 115(4):483–490

[48] Meditations for Pelvic Health. Nari Clemons. Audio CD

[49] Miller JM, Ashton-Miller JA, DeLancey JOL. A pelvic muscle precontraction can reduce cough-related urine loss in selected women with mild SUI. J Am Geriatr Soc. 1998; 46: 870–874

[50] National Association for Continence X

[51] O'Dwyer M. My Pelvic Flaw. Preventing Pelvic floor Problems Throughout Life. Redsok Publishing; 2007

[52] Pauls J, Shelly E. Applying Guide to Physical Therapist Practice to women's health. J Section Women's Health. 1999; 23 (3):8–12

[53] Peruchini D, DeLancey JOL. Functional anatomy of the pelvic floor and lower urinary tract. In: Baussler K, Shussler B, Burgio KL, Moore KH, Norton PA, Stanton S, eds. Pelvic Floor Re-education. 2nd ed. London, UK: Springer; 2008

[54] Retzky SS, Rogers RM, Jr. Urinary incontinence in women. Clin Symp. 1995; 47(3):2–32

[55] Richardson C, Jull G, Hodges P, Hides J. Therapeutic Exercises for Spinal Segmental Stabilization in Low Back Pain. Philadelphia: Churchill Livingstone; 1999

[56] Sapsford R. Rehabilitation of pelvic floor muscles utilizing trunk stabilization. Man Ther. 2004; 9(1):3–12

[57] Sapsford RR, Hodges PW, Richardson CA, Cooper DH, Markwell SJ, Jull GA. Co-activation of the abdominal and pelvic floor muscles during voluntary exercises. Neurourol Urodyn. 2001; 20(1):31–42

[58] Sawatzky R, Liu-Ambrose T, Miller WC, Marra CA. Physical activity as a mediator of the impact of chronic conditions on quality of life in older adults. Health Qual Life Outcomes. 2007; 5:68

[59] Schachter CL, Stalker CA, Teram E. Toward sensitive practice: issues for physical therapists working with survivors of childhood sexual abuse. Phys Ther. 1999; 79(3):248–261, discussion 262–269

[60] Schuh I. Bindegewebsmassage. Stuttgart: Gustav Fischer Verlag; 1986

[61] Schultz SE, Kopec JA. Impact of chronic conditions. Health Rep. 2003; 14(4):41–53

[62] Shah JP, Thaker N, Heimur J, Aredo JV, Sikdar S, Gerber L. Myofascial trigger points then and now: a historical and scientific perspective. PM R. 2015; 7(7): 746–761

[63] Sherburn M, Murphy CA, Carroll S, Allen TJ, Galea MP. Investigation of transabdominal real-time ultrasound to visualise the muscles of the pelvic floor. Aust J Physiother. 2005; 51(3):167–170

[64] Smith MD, Russell A, Hodges PW. Disorders of breathing and continence have a stronger association with back pain than obesity and physical activity. Aust J Physiother. 2006; 52(1):11–16

[65] Smith RP. Gynecology in Primary Care. Baltimore: William & Wilkins; 1997:501–516

[66] Steege JF, Metzger DA, Levy BS. Chronic Pelvic Pain. Philadelphia: WB Saunders; 1998

[67] Tanzberger R. Incontinence. In: Carrière B, ed. The Swiss Ball. Berlin-New York: Springer Verlag; 1998: 327–358

[68] Travell JG, Simons DG, eds. Myofascial Pain and Dysfunction: The Trigger Point Manual. Vol. 2. The Lower Extremities. Baltimore, MD: Williams & Wilkins; 1992

[69] Van Kampen M, De Weerdt W, Van Poppel H, Baert L. Urinary incontinence following transurethral, transvesical and radical prostatectomy. Retrospective study of 489 patients. Acta Urol Belg. 1997; 65(4):1–7

[70] Versprille-Fischer ES. Inkontinenz und Beckenbodendysfunktion. Berlin: Ullstein Mosby; 1997

[71] Von Gontard A. Einnässen im Kindesalter. Stuttgart: Thieme; 2001

[72] Wagner TH, Hu TW. Economic costs of urinary incontinence in 1995. Urology. 1998; 51(3):355–361

[73] Weiss JM. Pelvic floor myofascial trigger points: manual therapy for interstitial cystitis and the urgency-frequency syndrome. J Urol. 2001; 166(6):2226–2231

[74] Wesselmann U, Burnett AL, Heinberg LJ. The urogenital and rectal pain syndromes. Pain. 1997; 73(3):269–294

[75] Wise D, Anderson RU. A Headache in the Pelvis: A New Understanding and Treatment for Prostatitis and Chronic Pelvic Pain Syndromes. 6th ed. National Center for Pelvic Pain Research; 2018

Glossary

Antagonist: Muscle that opposes the movement of the prime mover (the agonist).

Autonomic nervous system: Involuntary nervous system with sympathetic fibers that inhibit and parasympathetic fibers that stimulate. Important for metabolic and physiological responses.

Brainstem: Contains the medulla oblongata, pons, and midbrain and is positioned below the brain, an extension of the spinal cord.

Catheter: Instrument placed into the urethra to drain urine from the bladder.

Cerebellum: Part of the brain that gathers information from different systems to determine adjustments of the muscle contraction, timing, coordination, and precision for the task intended.

Cervical spine: Section of the spine that forms part of the neck.

Coccygodynia: Pain in the area of the tail bone usually involving the pubococcygeus muscle.

Coccyx: Tail bone.

Colon: Section of the large intestine.

Colon massage: Massage that helps move the bowel (feces) in the colon.

Cone: Cone-shaped vaginal weights.

Connective-tissue massage: Treatment technique developed by Dicke and Teirich-Leube of Germany. Type of massage using reflex zones of the connective tissue between skin and muscle; can contribute to balancing the autonomic nervous system.

Continence: Ability to control bladder or bowel so that there is no involuntary loss of urine, feces, or gas.

Contraction of a muscle fiber: The muscle fibers shorten while actively moving.

Cortex, cerebral cortex: Gray matter of the brain above the brainstem.

Cystitis: Inflammatory condition of the bladder often as a result of infection.

Detrusor: Bladder muscle.

Diaphragm (pulmonary diaphragm): Dome-shaped muscle behind the rib cage, important for abdominal breathing.

Diuretics: Medications or foods that lead to increased urine output.

Dysfunction: Not functioning correctly.

Dyspareunia: Pain during penile penetration of intercourse.

Eccentric muscle contraction: Forced lengthening of a muscle tendon complex while contracting the muscle.

Endopelvic fascia: Fascia covering and supporting the organs of the pelvis, containing ligaments, smooth muscles, veins, arteries, nerves, and collagen.

Erectile dysfunction: Difficulty achieving erection of the penis.

Extensor muscles: Muscles that extend body parts and contribute to an upright posture.

Fascia: Connecting tissue, lining.

Fast muscle fibers: Muscle fibers that can react quickly, for example, when coughing or sneezing.

Feces: Bowel or excrement (waste) produced and expelled from the intestine.

Flexor muscles: Muscles used to bend joints.

Gastrointestinal: Relating to stomach and intestine.

Incontinence: Inability to hold urine, can also be related to feces.

Innervate: Supplying with a nerve. A nerve innervates muscles.

Interstitial cystitis: Painful bladder condition of unknown origin resulting in inflammation.

Levator ani muscle: Muscle considered the "lifter of the anus." It forms the pelvic diaphragm. The following muscles are part of the levator ani.
- *Iliococcygeus:* Extends between the ilium and the coccyx.
- *Coccygeus:* The tail-wagging muscle in animals. It does not lift the anus.
- *Pubococcygeus:* Extends between the pubic bones and the tail bone.
- *Puborectalis:* Originates at the pubic bones and passes around the rectum. It is part of the pubococcygeus and assists in providing continence of stool.
- *Pubovaginalis:* Part of the puborectalis that passes around the vagina.

- *Levator prostatae:* Lifter of the prostate gland in men.
- *Pubourethralis:* Supports the middle part of the urethra.

Limbic system: Area in the brain responsible for memory, motivation, and emotions.

Lumbar spine: The region of the low back.

Micturition: Emptying of the bladder.

Micturition centers: Centers in the spinal cord and brainstem coordinating emptying of the bladder.

Mixed incontinence: Mixture of stress and urge incontinence.

Motor learning: Learning a new movement task, aiming to perform it efficiently and skillfully, and to execute it at normal speed.

Neuron: Nerve cell.

Nocturia: Having to get up at night to urinate.

Nocturnal enuresis: Bed-wetting at night.

Overactive bladder: Condition that causes urgency with urination.

Overflow incontinence: Normal emptying of the bladder is prevented by an obstruction to the outflow resulting in leakage.

Palpate: Feel by touching with the fingers.

Pelvic diaphragm: Inner layer of muscles (levator ani, pubococcygeus, puborectalis, pubovaginalis, and iliococcygeus) which are part of the pelvic floor.

Physical: Relating to the body.

Postural alignment: The ability to align pelvis, trunk, and neck and head effortlessly in a straight line, enabling good posture. Requires the muscles of the body to be the proper length.

Prompted voiding: Reminding a person at regular intervals to empty the bladder.

Prostate: Gland surrounding the urethra in men which produces sperm.

Prostatectomy: Surgical removal of part or all of the prostate gland.

Prostatitis: Inflammation of the prostate gland.

Proximal: Close to the center of the body.

Pubic bones: Two bones forming the junction at the front arch of the pelvis. The bladder rests behind and below the pubic bones when empty.

Part of the levator ani muscle arises from the pubic bones.

Pudendal nerve: Innervates all the pelvic floor muscles, also supplies feeling to the area of the pelvic floor.

Pulmonary diaphragm: See diaphragm.

Quick flicks: Fast muscle contractions.

Rectum: Part of the large intestine, referring to the "straight" section leading to the anal canal.

Rotation: Turning movement.

Sacroiliac joint: Joint formed by the bones of the sacrum and the ilium. There are many muscles influencing the joint, but none connecting these two bones. Pain in the region is common after a fall on the buttock or when missing a step or slipping.

Sacrum: Triangular bone of fused vertebrae, sits between the two iliac bones of the pelvis.

Sensory system: Part of the nervous system that deals with feeling (sensation).

Slow muscle fibers: Muscle fibers that sustain the muscle tone for a long time.

Smooth muscles: Muscles under involuntary control that do not fatigue easily, such as the heart or the bladder muscle.

Stress incontinence: Involuntary loss of urine during instances of increased physical stress such as coughing, sneezing, or running.

Sympathetic nerve: Nerve fibers, component of the autonomic system, that inhibit and help regulate the vegetative functions.

Symphysis pubis: Region at the front part of the pelvis where the pubic bones of each side form a joint.

Thoracic spine: The section of the spine of the thorax below the neck and above the low back.

Timed voiding: Placing a person at regular intervals on a toilet to avoid incontinence.

Tonus or tone: Tension or relative stiffness of a muscle. The pelvic floor muscles have a high muscle tone to provide continence at night.

Urethra: Canal through which urine is expelled from the bladder, approximately 4 cm long in women. In men it passes through the prostate gland and the penis and is much longer.

Urge incontinence: Involuntary bladder contractions increasing the frequency and desire to empty the bladder, sometimes leading to involuntary loss of urine.

Urogenital diaphragm: Outer layer of pelvic floor muscles consisting of:

- *Deep transverse perineal muscle:* Helps provide continence of urine.
- *Superficial transverse perineal muscle:* Supports the action of the deep transverse perineal muscle.
- *Bulbocavernosus (also called bulbospongiosus):* Important for sexual function, assisting in the erection of the penis and squirting the last drop of urine out at the end of urination. In female it contributes to the erection of the clitoris. It also constricts the opening of the vagina.
- *Ischiocavernosus:* Enhances penile erection in men; in women it sustains the erection of the clitoris during sexual activity.
- *Anal sphincter:* Ring-shaped muscle at the end of the digestive tract. Provides continence.

Uterus: Pear-shaped muscle; part of the female reproductive system.

Vagina: Outer part of the sexual organs of women, leading to the uterus.

Vaginismus: Inability to relax the muscles of the vaginal opening during penetration.

Vegetative nervous system: See autonomic nervous system.

Viscera: Inner organs of the body and pelvis.

Visceral mobilization: Manual treatment to allow the inner organs to return to their normal position.

Visualization: Imagining a task or a movement.

Void: To empty the bladder.

Index

Note: Page numbers set **bold** or *italic* indicate headings or figures, respectively.